Alzheimer's Disease
&
the Dementias

Alzheimer's Disease & the Dementias

AN ALTERNATIVE PERSPECTIVE

Based on the Readings of Edgar Cayce

David McMillin, M.A.

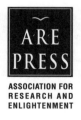

ARE PRESS

ASSOCIATION FOR
RESEARCH AND
ENLIGHTENMENT

A.R.E. Press • Virginia Beach • Virginia

DISCLAIMER: This book is directed primarily to health care profession-als who are interested in alternative perspectives on the causes and treatment of mental illness. This book should not be regarded as a guide to self-diagnosis or self-treatment. The cooperation of a qualified health care professional is essential if one wishes to apply the principles and techniques discussed in this book.

Copyright © 1994
by David McMillin
1st Printing, July 1994 by Lifeline Press

Alzheimer's Disease & The Dementias
3rd Printing, September 1997 by A.R.E. Press

Printed in the U.S.A.

A.R.E. Press
Sixty-Eighth & Atlantic Avenue
P.O. Box 656
Virginia Beach, VA 23451-0656

Library of Congress Cataloging-in-Publication Data
McMillin, David.
Alzheimer's disease and the dementias : an alternative perspec-tive based on the readings of Edgar Cayce / by David McMillin.
    p.   cm.
Originally published: Virginia Beach, Va. : Lifeline Press, ©1994.
Includes bibliographical references.
ISBN 0-87604-380-5
1. Alzheimer's disease—Alternative treatment. 2. Dementia—Al-ternative treatment. 3. Cayce, Edgar, 1877-1945. Edgar Cayce read-ings. I. Title.
RC523.M42   1997
616.8'3106—dc21   96-54001

Cover design by Richard Boyle

CONTENTS

Introduction

◆————————

AMERICA IS ENTERING an era of health care crisis. While politicians debate alternatives, insurance companies and hospitals feel the pressure to find less expensive and more efficient ways of doing business. Financially beleaguered citizens are often forced to forego medical services as the cost of treatment continues to rise. At all levels, there appears to be a growing concern that our health care system is failing and may eventually collapse.

We are offered a foretaste (although for most of us second hand) of this impending dilemma via the current AIDS crisis. As a society and as individuals it is easy to become preoccupied (or even terrorized) by the possibility of contamination by this menacing virus which incapacitates our immune system.

However, AIDS is only a forerunner of the difficulties before us. There is increasing evidence of a more ominous crisis. We are becoming more aware of diseases which preferentially afflict the aged, a group of disorders called the dementias.

In particular, tremendous resources are being focused on the most widely recognized of the dementias—Alzheimer's disease. Unlike the AIDS dilemma, our present level of understanding does not allow us to forego the risk of Alzheimer's dementia by simply abstaining from certain behaviors or taking precautions when risk is inevitable. The bottom line is that we are all at risk and remain at risk until we can achieve significant advances in the treatment and/ or prevention of this form of dementia. We will discuss some of the staggering statistics associated with the impending Alzheimer's epidemic in Chapter One.

I am not alone and certainly not the first to ring the alarm concerning this devastating illness. However, my angle is definitely unique and I assure you that this is not a doom and gloom tale. To the contrary, it is a statement of cautious optimism tempered by a realistic assessment of the seriousness of our predicament and the limitations of our resources.

Of course, like ostriches we can stick our heads in the proverbial sand. Or in a more typically American fashion, we can optimistically hold down the fort of modern medical health care and wait for the clinical cavalry to come to our rescue.

Adopting this strategy, our hopes would have to ride heavily on medical research. Although we strongly support such research, we must also be realistic and look at the track record of science in regard to chronic, degenerative disorders. It is certainly a mixed bag. Having invested years of research and billions of dollars, we have failed to conquer a multitude of major illnesses such as multiple sclerosis, muscular dystrophy, cancer, cardiovascular disorders, arthritis, etc.

Certainly, gains have been made. This is especially true in disorders involving serious mental symptoms. However, most of the primary therapeutic advances in the field of major mental illness have resulted from serendipity. The right person happened to be in the right place at a fortuitous moment.

For example, the discovery of the antipsychotic properties of the phenothiazines (such as Thorazine) can be traced back to the French physician Henri Laborit. He was looking for a drug to prevent a drop in blood pressure during surgery. Although the drug he used failed in that respect, it did have noticeable sedative effects. Subsequent research by French psychiatrists was by trial and error— they gave the drug to persons suffering a wide range of disorders to see if it had any effect. The medication had potent calming effects on agitated psychotic patients and thus: "The first powerful drug available to treat serious mental illness was discovered in much the same way as was penicillin: by accident. The discovery was the happy consequence of a chance finding being observed by a person with a fertile mind who could recognize its larger implications." The preceding observation was noted by Nancy Andreasen, M.D., Ph.D., a leading researcher in the field of mental illness.

The efficacy of lithium carbonate, a naturally occurring salt useful in the treatment of mood disorders such as manic-depression, was also a fortuitous accident. Its therapeutic potential was discovered by an Australian researcher seeking a neutral solution to serve as a control substance in experiments with rats. Fortunately, he was astute enough to notice that the substance, intended to have no effect, actually affected the rats' behavior in a specific and useful manner. He had a difficult time convincing his colleagues to give lithium a try—it had been used in previous experiments with humans and its propensity for toxicity had resulted in several deaths. Eventually, its therapeutic value was acknowledged and now is widely used by the medical profession in treating mood disorders.

Finally, the use of "monoamine-oxidase inhibitors" (or MAOIs, a class of drugs used to treat depression) can also be traced to a lucky side effect. One of the MAOIs is an antibiotic used to treat tuberculosis. Clinicians noted that the drug helped to relieve the depression which also plagued the patients. Subsequent trial and error experiments further refined the applications of anti-depressant drugs.

Compared to these serendipities, the list of major therapeutic breakthroughs resulting from a concentrated study of a mental illness and thorough understanding of the problem is meager. The fact is, we *still* don't know for sure what causes these disorders or exactly how the drugs suppress the undesirable symptoms. So the image of successful research (i.e., a team of knowledgable researchers who produce an effective treatment based on a thorough understanding of the condition—and millions of dollars in government funding) is not necessarily accurate or comforting.

With this in mind, we should remain open to any source of information which offers a reasonable possibility of making a contribution. A premise of this book is that the psychic readings of Edgar Cayce are such a source. Naturally, readers will have to judge for themselves the plausibility of this material. No attempt will be made to convince or convert anyone to this perspective. The readings themselves acknowledge the necessity of seeking such information:

No one should be . . . coerced. No one should be sought. But EVERYONE should be given the opportunity that would sincerely seek. (254-96)

Thus, the purpose of this book is to make the information readily available to anyone seeking and open to this source. This work is merely presented as a service to those desiring an alternative perspective on the treatment of dementia.

It will not appeal to most. We are an impatient society spoiled by the illusions of miracle cures. We tend to seek an easy and quick, non-involved remedy for our ills—a pill, injection, or some other straightforward medical intervention.

The perspective presented in this book is not so detached. The therapeutic process requires a great deal from the caregivers who implement it. However, it also has tremendous potential.

This book is directed primarily to the families and support persons dealing with dementias such as Alzheimer's disease. It is nontechnical in style and seeks to make the Cayce material accessible to those who are interested in alternative perspectives on this disorder.

This book does not pretend to present a cure. Yet, the readings do offer some extremely optimistic possibilities for those who patiently and consistently apply the recommendations. Thus, this information will be presented—but not without acknowledgment of how extremely difficult such a process is.

I will not attempt to address the causes and treatment of dementia in any deep or scholarly fashion. I will leave that to the clinical researchers. However, I will include some references in Chapter One regarding demographics. The projected statistics for the dementias (and especially Alzheimer's) are so consequential that I feel it best that readers have the opportunity to follow up on this literature if they desire. Therefore, I have referenced some of the more imposing data concerning future rates of occurrence and the projected financial burden this will incur.

I have also referenced all of the selections from the Cayce readings. Recognizing the need for confidentiality, each reading is assigned a number corresponding to the person or group requesting information. The identifying number is followed by another number designating the sequence of the reading. For example, a reading cited as 182-6 indicates that this reading is the sixth in a series of readings for an individual or group designated as 182. Although many of the early readings were not recorded, over 14,000 were stenographically transcribed and have been preserved by the Association for Research and Enlightenment (A.R.E.) in Virginia Beach, Virginia. Readers seeking a deeper understanding of this material may pursue their interest at the A.R.E. Library—it is open to the public on a daily basis.

This book may be viewed as an introduction to the dementias from a unique, alternative perspective. The Appendix contains a list of resources including books and articles for persons wishing further information on the subject. The chapters which follow merely present a way of looking at the problem which may help those who have to deal with it on a daily basis. At this level of daily involvement, relief of symptoms and delay of degeneration is a significant contribution. The readings may have something to offer in this area.

The suggestions are "low-tech" in nature and for the most part can be provided at home (if such is the desire of those providing care). The assistance of health care professionals is required for some treatments. However these therapies are not beyond the resources of most families. For example, an osteopath or chiropractor may be able to provide the primary treatments recommended in the readings. The services of a massage therapist may also be helpful (even this therapy may be provided by a family member willing to learn some basic techniques).

This book is also about attitudes—how to think about the problems posed by a chronic debilitating illness. How to make the best of a bad situation. The psychological and spiritual aspects of treatment are important and will be emphasized.

This approach deals with all levels of human experience and is especially helpful in addressing the *meaning* of illness. Disease can be a pathway to growth in consciousness. In this sense, dementia may offer an opportunity for soul growth for the suffering individual as well as family, friends, and professional caregivers.

1

Our Dilemma

◆————————

BEFORE LAUNCHING INTO the psychic readings of Edgar Cayce, it will be helpful to get an overview of our topic. This preliminary survey will define key terms, explain important concepts and theories, and provide some statistics which will convey the seriousness of the impending medical crisis.

Thus, this brief chapter will set the stage for a consideration of Edgar Cayce's alternative perspective of the dementias. A basic understanding of the facts, as they are currently discerned, will provide a baseline with which to evaluate the potential contribution of the readings.

What Is Dementia?

Dementia is a medical term referring to a deterioration of mental functioning due to progressive organic disease of the brain. Persons suffering from dementia typically experience loss of intellectual abilities such as memory, language use, and the ability to learn, solve problems, and make judgments. In its more severe forms, dementia may also produce disorientation, hallucinations, and paranoia. Social functioning is impaired and emotional responses may be atypical or inappropriate. For example, irritability and agitation may be present with occasional verbal and physical aggression toward family or caregivers.

Family members often describe the deterioration of a demented relative as a gradual death—as a loss of the higher qualities of the mind which distinguish us as human beings. This is an ironic observation since dementia often strikes while the individual still has good physical health.

Eventually, even the body succumbs. Dementia is a leading cause of death among U.S. adults. (1)

Dementia is an acquired illness (as contrasted to disorders present at birth such as mental retardation). Alzheimer's disease (a widely publicized dementia which we will look at more closely later in this chapter) accounts for about 50 to 60 percent of all cases of dementia. Vascular disease contributes around 10 to 20 percent.

Dementia may be caused by a multitude of factors including brain injuries, nutritional deficiencies, epilepsy, infections, hormone disorders, and drug effects. The list of causes is extensive and still growing with at least sixty known factors or conditions which can lead to dementia. There is still much to be learned about the causes of dementia. Even extensive postmortem examinations fail to reveal the cause of dementia in about five percent of all cases.

The outcome in cases of dementia is variable. Many dementias are reversible—that is, if a correct diagnosis is made and appropriate treatment provided, the deterioration can be halted or even reversed. This is particularly true in cases of malnutrition and vitamin deficiencies. Because many elderly people develop poor eating habits due to limited finances, difficulty in chewing, and other factors which often affect dietary choices, this area should be thoroughly assessed by the health care professional making the diagnosis.

Dementia is closely linked to the aging process—as we become older, we are at greater risk for developing dementia. Currently there are approximately two million patients suffering from dementia in this country. As the "baby boom" generation moves into its golden years, this number will increase dramatically. Based on current rates of occurrence (that is, if there are no major breakthroughs in the treatment or prevention of dementia), in the year 2040 there will be approximately 7.4 million Americans suffering from dementia. (2)

The total cost of caring for demented persons runs into the billions of dollars (many estimates focus on the $25-$30 billion range).(1) If the projected increase in frequency is accurate, the financial burden of providing medical services could bankrupt the health service system of our country.

In the past, dementia was viewed as a normal consequence of the aging process. Just as the body tended to lose its strength and suppleness with the passage of time, aging was also thought to naturally result in brain degeneration and decline in mental abilities. This view was (and still is to some extent) reflected in the term senility. Although in our daily lives we commonly associate senility with aging, technically it is not a useful medical term. With the increased understanding of the role of the dementias in the aging process, senility has fallen from favor. It is simply too vague in its implications to be useful to health care professionals.

Only a few years ago, senility was employed for diagnostic purposes. To understand how the change in medical terminology took place, we must look back almost a century. In 1907, Dr. Alois Alzheimer published research findings based on a case study which indicated that biological deterioration was linked to the psychological symptoms of certain forms of dementia. This important demonstration of biological causation was a crucial step in recognizing that mental illness can have a physical origin. His description of the tangled and degenerated nerve fibers clearly established the biological dimension of a process then labeled senility.

The curious feature of Alzheimer's case study was that the patient was only fifty-one years old. The woman's age was far too young to be considered normal for such extensive degeneration. Alzheimer believed that he had discovered a separate illness occurring before old age. Therefore he called the disease presenile dementia—dementia before old age.

Although his findings were controversial, his diagnostic category was eventually accepted. An arbitrary age limit (sixty-five) was chosen. Sixty-five years of age was thought to reflect the age at which "normal" senility began. Thus, cases of dementia of unknown causation before the age of sixty-five were diagnosed as presenile dementia, while those sixty-five or older were considered senile dementia.

This bit of historical information is very important to our consideration of Edgar Cayce's perspective in Chapter Two. Alzheimer's disease was not a formal diagnostic category during Cayce's lifetime.

As one would expect, when he did use diagnostic labels, Cayce tended to use terms commonly in use among the health care professionals of his era.

Therefore, many of the readings which appear to be describing Alzheimer type pathology simply mention senility as the problem. Apparently, he did recognize the generally accepted medical distinction between presenile and senile dementia. For example, he used the term "premature senility" to distinguish dementia with an earlier onset. However in terms of treatment, he adopted a position more in line with modern medical thinking. He tended to ignore the distinction by treating them as one disorder. We will continue this discussion of the problem of diagnostic classification in the readings in later chapters.

Until the late 1960s, arteriosclerosis ("hardening of the arteries") was viewed as the major cause of senile dementia. This view changed when researchers established that large amounts of fatty deposits could be found in the brain's arterial walls of both demented and normal elderly individuals. Furthermore, approximately half of the brains of persons suffering from dementia showed no signs of significant arteriosclerosis. So, while some cases of dementia could be attributed to vascular disease, it was not viewed as a major factor.

Research also clarified the nature of the brain lesions in both presenile and senile dementia. The brain pathology was identical. Apparently, the age distinction of sixty-five years was not relevant in making a diagnosis. Medical terminology was modified to reflect this recognition. The two groups were combined and called dementia of the Alzheimer type (DAT).

With further research, this nomenclature could change again. While medical science tends to focus on diseases as specific conditions (with specific causes and specific cures), there is a growing recognition of the complexity of major illnesses such as Alzheimer's dementia. This is sometimes referred to as "nonspecificity." Nonspecificity is an important concept in the readings of Edgar Cayce and we will be looking more closely at its implications for both causation and treatment in subsequent chapters. For now, it is only necessary to grasp that Alzheimer's dementia may not be a single illness. Dr. Leonard L. Heston and associates have noted: " . . . that widespread etiologic heterogeneity exists in nature and that eventually evidence will be found to support extensive subdivision of DAT [dementia of the Alzheimer type]." (3) In other words, this dementia may consist of a group of related diseases with different causes and course of illness which result in the characteristic destruction of brain tissue associated with Alzheimer's dementia.

The possibility that a variety of factors may be involved in Alzheimer's dementia is apparent from the list of suspected causes. We will briefly consider the most prominent of these suspects.

Some Possible Causes of Alzheimer's Disease

While the cause of Alzheimer's dementia is unknown, there are several theories which have attracted considerable attention. Researchers have proposed that it may result from *viral infections* which attack brain cells and cause slow deterioration of nerve tissue. Parallels have been drawn to two similar diseases of the brain (kuru and Creutzfeldt-Jakob disease) which are known to result from viral infection. Scientists at the National Institutes of Health have explored the possibility of a viral link in Alzheimer's dementia by taking brain cells from deceased victims and placing the diseased cells in laboratory dishes containing normal cells. In certain cases, the diseased tissues appeared to cause the normal cells to die.

In related experiments, diseased cells were injected into the brains of chimpanzees. Two of the six experimental animals developed a progressive neurological disease.

Unfortunately, further research failed to support the results of either of these types of experiment. As we shall see, this pattern of apparent initial breakthrough followed by failure of experimental confirmation is common in research of this disorder.

For example, it is widely accepted that aluminum toxicity can produce brain degeneration similar to the lesions of Alzheimer's dementia. Findings on experimental animals have shown that injections of aluminum compounds produce neurological tangles in the brain similar to those found in Alzheimer's dementia. Early in the 1970s, researchers at the University of Toronto explored a possible connection between aluminum and Alzheimer's dementia. Their findings were dramatic. Autopsies of brains from patients who had been diagnosed as Alzheimer's dementia contained as much as 30 times more aluminum than normal brains.

However, subsequent research has clouded these findings. Investigators at the University of Kentucky failed to find significant amounts of aluminum in the brains of Alzheimer's patients even though these individuals had spent a lifetime drinking local water containing high levels of aluminum.

So we are left with the question of whether aluminum toxicity might be a cause of Alzheimer's dementia. This is a particularly fascinating aspect of the Alzheimer's puzzle since the Edgar Cayce readings were cautioning against the use of aluminum cooking utensils decades before researchers became aware of its potential link with a major brain disease.

Currently, scientists are focusing a great deal of attention on the genetic aspects of Alzheimer's dementia. Research indicates that children of parents with the disease have a 50 percent chance of developing the illness. Furthermore, these individuals are more likely to exhibit the symptoms much earlier with a more rapid progression in the degenerative process.

The genetic link is further emphasized by studies connecting Alzheimer's dementia with Down's syndrome. Down's syndrome is a developmental disorder in which a child is born mentally retarded. It is caused by a flaw in the genetic material of the afflicted person. These individuals have an extra copy of chromosome 21.

Persons with Down's syndrome who survive beyond the age of forty typically suffer brain degeneration similar to Alzheimer's dementia. Furthermore, the frequency of Down's syndrome is 10 times higher among families of persons who experience early-onset Alzheimer's dementia.

As persuasive as the genetic studies are, we should be cautious in interpreting their meaning. Genetics is not likely to hold all the answers to the Alzheimer's puzzle. For example, even with identical twins, one twin may develop the disease while the other does not. Obviously, there are additional factors at work here. Perhaps certain genetic factors can make an individual vulnerable to developing Alzheimer's dementia while other factors (such as environment or lifestyle) can increase a person's vulnerability. We will address this possibility in a later chapter which focuses on preventing dementia.

Direct brain insult is another possible cause of Alzheimer's dementia. It is known that persons whose brains have been seriously jarred or who have experienced repeated blows to the head may develop the symptoms of Alzheimer's. For example, prizefighters who have received numerous punches to the head over a period of years may develop "boxer's dementia," an irreversible dementia with symptoms and brain degeneration very similar to Alzheimer's.

Glandular abnormalities have been linked to Alzheimer's dementia. Researchers at Duke University have found a significantly higher frequency of prior thyroid disease in women patients suffering from Alzheimer's than in control subjects. Furthermore, studies at the University of Minnesota suggest that the immune system may play a part in Alzheimer's dementia.

These findings result from statistical analysis of biographical data collected from patients and control subjects. Correlating life history patterns with specific biological pathology has been more difficult. One of the most promising models links certain forms of Alzheimer's dementia with "disorders comprising the thyroid-gastricadrenal-thymic autoimmune syndrome." (3) It is likely that future research will uncover more extensive connections between glandular dysfunction and Alzheimer's dementia.

We have looked at only a few of the most prominent theories explaining the causes of Alzheimer's dementia. New hypotheses and variations on the older theories are being proposed continually. The bottom line at this point in time is that we really do not know what causes Alzheimer's dementia.

Symptoms of Alzheimer's Dementia

Like many of the other dementias, Alzheimer's disease results in the progressive loss of "higher" functions such as thinking, reasoning, and memory. It destroys the distinctive qualities of mentality which make us human.

The deterioration is usually gradual, beginning with mild symptoms (such as forgetfulness of minor things like phone numbers or dental appointments). This decline is often accompanied by difficulty in learning new information. As the nervous system becomes more incapacitated, patients may have difficulty controlling their bodies or moving smoothly. Emotional problems commonly develop. The degeneration in functioning may produce deep depression, crying spells, or temper tantrums.

The Demographics of Alzheimer's Dementia

Nursing homes contain many cases of Alzheimer's dementia. Researchers estimate that as many as half of the patients in nursing homes are suffering from it. (1) Furthermore, it is the fourth leading cause of death among older people. (4)

The number of cases of Alzheimer's dementia has increased dramatically during this century. It is currently 10 times more frequent than it was during the first decade of the twentieth century when it was identified by Dr. Alzheimer. By the end of the century the number of cases will likely increase by an additional 60 percent. (2)

Ironically, this alarming increase is due, in large measure, to the success of medical science in extending the human lifespan. Because people are living longer, the number of elderly people at risk for Alzheimer's dementia is greater.

Consider these facts: 9 out of 10 persons afflicted with the disorder are over 65 years of age. It occurs in about 1 percent of all persons between the ages of 65 and 74 years of age, 7 percent in those individuals 75 to 84 years old, and 25 percent in the population who are 85 years or older. (2)

Since the average age of persons in our society is steadily increasing and will dramatically accelerate with the aging of the "baby boom" generation, we may soon find ourselves in the midst of an Alzheimer's dementia epidemic. Some researchers and family members affected by the disease have suggested that we are already experiencing such an epidemic. Some doctors refer to Alzheimer's dementia as the "disease of the century." With the increasing threat posed by the AIDS virus, this unflattering designation is certainly debatable.

However, if we are unable to make major breakthroughs in the prevention and/or treatment of Alzheimer's dementia in the next couple of decades, it will certainly deserve the title of "disease of the 21st century." If the present trend continues unabated, by the year 2034 the incidence of Alzheimer's dementia in the American population will more than triple. (2)

By the year 2040, there will be 7.4 million Americans stricken with dementia (mostly suffering from Alzheimer's dementia). In such a scenario, half the American population would suffer from Alzheimer's or some other form of dementia before they die. (2) As it stands today, at least 10 percent of the readers of this book will eventually develop some form of dementia.

The National Institutes of Health estimates that Alzheimer's dementia costs about thirty billion dollars each year, the bulk of the expense going to institutionalization of chronic Alzheimer patients. (4) The financial burden is likely to double or triple in the next thirty to fifty years as the "baby boom" generation advances into old age. (1) Unless medical science can produce a major breakthrough in the prevention or treatment of Alzheimer's dementia, America will soon be confronted with an age-related medical emergency, spearheaded by an Alzheimer's dementia epidemic.

There is a natural tendency to be overwhelmed by such incredibly large numbers stretching forward into an uncertain future. Furthermore, researchers and experts in this field sometimes add to our confusion by quibbling over specifics of the demographics we have just reviewed. However, there does seem to be a consensus on the general trend we are experiencing. Dementia is presently a very serious health care problem confronting us all, individually and collectively. The problem will likely become significantly more difficult in the next few decades.

The Course of the Disease

While the course of Alzheimer's dementia may vary in individual cases, the ultimate prognosis is the same—incurable with progressive decline in functioning at all levels. Premature death can be expected, either directly as the result of the organic deterioration or by related syndromes which are caused or exacerbated by the dementia.

Treatment of Alzheimer's Dementia

Whereas some of the other dementias are treatable (and even curable if the cause is detected and amenable to therapy), the therapeutic options available for Alzheimer's dementia are mainly limited to adaptive measures. That is, when faced with an incurable progressive illness, the usual strategy is to minimize the effects on patient and family. Rather than directly treating the illness, therapy involves adapting to it.

These adaptive measures range from behavioral interventions (which organize and simplify daily activities) to general physical interventions (such as basic health maintenance). For example, basic health maintenance might involve bowel regulation. Constipation is often a problem for persons suffering from Alzheimer's dementia. Dietary changes, drinking adequate water, and the use of laxatives can help to address this problem.

Individual counseling and support groups for caregivers are two additional forms of therapy which can facilitate the process of adaptation. For many families, institutional care (such as nursing homes) represent the final stage of adaptation.

Research has yielded some promising medicinal therapies over the years. Unfortunately, these drugs have not produced consistent results under the rigors of scientific standards of confirmation. Consequently, the therapeutic effectiveness of drug therapy for Alzheimer's dementia is controversial.

Antidepressant medications are commonly prescribed for persons with Alzheimer's dementia since depression is one of the most frequent and debilitating symptoms associated with the disease. Again, however, these drugs do not directly treat the dementia—they are only adaptive measures intended to provide limited symptomatic relief.

Summary

The personal devastation caused by dementia is extreme—it destroys the essence of our humanity, our mental processes. It is a progressive degeneration often taking years to complete its wrecking of the brain. This process unfolds as slow death, day by day, culminating in the disintegration of the person. This biological and psychological desolation typically parallels the toll taken on family resources—emotional and financial.

The social fallout from dementia may be just as devastating. As we live longer and the baby boom generation approaches the stage of life where risk of dementia is greatest, our social resources will be stretched to the limit—perhaps beyond the limit. Unless we can achieve major breakthroughs in the prevention and/or treatment of dementia (and particularly Alzheimer's dementia), we face an alarming future.

Although we recognize the causes of some of the dementias, we do not know what causes Alzheimer's dementia. However, this is a "hot" research area. Hopefully medical science can make major breakthroughs in understanding this disorder.

Likewise, medical science has not yet produced a cure for Alzheimer's dementia. New drugs are constantly being tested. Some medications appear to suppress certain symptoms in some individuals. However, there is no widely acknowledged treatment which is effective in halting or reversing the course of the illness.

Therefore, it behooves us to be open to alternative perspectives on the causes and treatment of the dementias. In the next chapter, we will be examining the psychic readings of Edgar Cayce—a remarkable source of information on this important subject.

2

An Alternative Perspective of Dementia

◆

EDGAR CAYCE GAVE many readings for persons suffering from various forms of dementia. In this chapter, I will provide some definitions and descriptions of Cayce's view of this group of neurological disorders. In order to clarify the distinctiveness of this approach, I will compare and contrast this point of view with modern medical concepts. Finally, I will provide real-life examples of Cayce's perspective in the form of case studies taken from the readings.

What Is Dementia?

The readings are in close agreement with modern medicine on the physical pathology of the dementias. Repeatedly, Edgar Cayce provided graphic descriptions of the nervous system deterioration indicative of these disorders. One almost gets the sense that Cayce used his consciousness as a modern researcher might use a high-tech probe or brain scan. Often, Cayce's perspective was from the inside of the body, moving freely among the organs and tissue. His portrayal of the delicate interactions within and between the nervous systems are particularly fascinating. We will be taking a closer look at these reports later in this chapter. For now, the important point is that from Cayce's perspective dementia involves a progressive degeneration of nerve tissue. Consider these brief excerpts from the readings which explicitly convey the physical pathology involved in dementia:

> Dementia in the act that the repressions are as magnified, and will eventually—without correction—bring the softening of cell tissue in brain itself. Hence we find there are periods when the body is not controlled by any reaction in self . . . unless corrections are made . . . we may expect a continued reaction . . . then the general breaking down of the gray portion of nerve tissue, nerve cell matter, in the body. (3997-1)

> . . . there are distresses caused in the coordination of the sympathetic and cerebrospinal nerve system produced by pressure in the lumbar and sacral region . . . [we need] the application of those properties as will bring for the replenishing of the white tissue in the nerve cells themselves—these, we find, would be aiding and bringing the nearer normal reaction, will these be taken in time, before the pressure produces the softening of the brain tissue itself; until there is dementia in its reaction. (5715-1)

> This, then, is the difference between an unbalanced condition in a mental reaction [a nervous breakdown] and that of dementia—which destroys the reaction in the plasm of the nerve as fixed from the blood supply itself . . . (386-1)

Many people are surprised by such graphic accounts of physical deterioration. Apparently, there is a strong expectation that psychic readings from such a renowned seer should emphasize the nonphysical (i.e., mental and spiritual) phases of the condition.

Certainly, this is not an unreasonable expectancy, for the readings do speak to the condition of the whole person. In fact, Edgar Cayce has been widely acclaimed as the "father of modern holistic medicine." This title derives from the readings' perspective of the human condition. According to this view, we are each triune beings consisting of body, mind, and spirit. The readings go so far as to talk of mental and spiritual bodies which coexist and connect with the physical body at definite anatomical centers within the physical body.

Coordination among these aspects of the self—the physical, mental, and spiritual—is essential for a normal functioning human experience. Incoordination among these aspects can manifest as a variety of illnesses, including the dementias.

Even when the readings consider a single aspect of the triune, for instance the physical, the emphasis is on taking a broader view of the body. This is even true in cases of dementia, where brain pathology is undeniable:

> Too little importance is too often given by those who would aid in bringing a normal force for a body suffering under even dementia, that relationship between the sympathetic and the cerebrospinal nervous systems . . . (5475-1)

So even in illnesses of the brain, the readings insisted on taking a broader perspective and looking at the peripheral systems—in this case, the nerves running within and along the spinal column.

The language of the readings can be a stumbling block in certain cases because the entranced Cayce utilized the medical terminology of his day. During the early decades of this century, the central nervous system (which includes the brain and spinal cord) was referred to as the cerebrospinal system. The autonomic nervous system was referred to as the sympathetic system. So if you encounter these terms in a reading, it may be helpful for you to translate cerebrospinal into its current equivalent—the central nervous system. Likewise, you may wish to think of the sympathetic system as the autonomic nervous system. This is a bit of an oversimplification since the readings present a much deeper appreciation of the way the nervous systems interact (and particularly the role of the sympathetic system). However, for purposes of our discussion this will suffice.

There are a couple of important reasons for expanding the discussion of dementia beyond the brain. First, the brain does not exist entirely in isolation from the rest of the body. True, it is surrounded by bone (the skull) and protected by a chemical boundary (the "blood-brain barrier") which allows in only those substances essential for brain functioning. However, the brain is constantly reliant upon the rest of the body for nourishment and removal of metabolic wastes.

The brain is also reliant upon the peripheral nervous systems for information about our external and internal environments. I am speaking here primarily of the sensory nervous system. If the sensory system is faulty, brain functioning will also be compromised. As computer programmers have noted—garbage in, garbage out.

Finally, because the readings insist that we are each triune beings or "ENTITIES," we might benefit from considering the interactions among these aspects of ourselves. For example, ponder the following excerpt which addresses the physical and mental dimensions of dementia:

> . . . for in almost every condition—even as in this [dementia]—there is found that the centers from which the radial forces of impulse by reaction of the mental body—that is, the sensory system—to the sympathetic forces, in those centers where they connect with the cerebrospinal—the cerebrospinal, then, is as the brain's reaction to the physical, or the material body; while those of the sympathetic system are more those of the reaction to the mental being, or the mental body; these must coordinate, that the reactions in a physical body bring about the proper reactions. (5475-1)

Note the references to the sensory and sympathetic nervous systems. Even while the brain is the primary focus of pathology, the peripheral nervous systems are important. The reading actually identifies these peripheral systems as embodying the "reaction to the mental being." In other words, the incoordination of the mental being (or mental body) with the brain's reaction is affected by the nerve connections along the spinal column and throughout the body. The deterioration of mental faculties (such as memory and intellect) are likewise linked to the coordination of the nerves at these important centers or plexus in the body.

In other readings involving dementia, the coordination of the spirit connection to the body was emphasized. In these cases, the glands (which Cayce regarded as "spiritual centers" within the body) was often dysfunctional in some manner.

Thus, the interface of mind and spirit with the body is regarded as quite literal—mind functioning primarily through the nervous systems and spirit manifesting through the glands. From this perspective, the intimate interaction between the nervous and glandular systems is emphasized. These systems work together to maintain the integrity of the whole self.

Consequently the readings digress from modern medicine on the meaning of disease and how physical degeneration is related to the broader context of the human experience. This context may be designated as holism, a term expressing the importance of considering all facets of human functioning.

Even strictly at the physical level, this alternative perspective has practical implications. The whole body is taken into consideration since mind and spirit manifest at various centers throughout the body. This is particularly significant with regard to the types of therapies which were most commonly suggested in the readings. We will explore these therapeutic implications in the next chapter. For now, we shall focus on some of the causes of dementia by looking at a few exemplary case studies from the readings.

Some Case Studies of Dementia

The Case of Mrs. [1553]

Mrs. [1553] was 71 years old when she received a series of 26 readings on her demented condition. A concerned son-in-law (Mr. [1561]) wrote to Edgar Cayce on April 17, 1938, stating that her:

> . . . "mind" remains not clear . . . The illness is commonly call[ed] "stroke"—and hardening of the arteries, plus chronic constipation . . . I do not know how to ask pertinent questions, but could her brain cells function, either "renewed in life" or compensatory cells take on the work . . . Now she has little control over her emotions—yet at times her mind seems clear and then it is [that] her thoughts return to "service" to others—as has been her life's experience . . .

This description is certainly indicative of dementia, possibly multi-infarct dementia resulting from stroke. Subsequent letters indicated that portions of the left side of her body were paralyzed and that her caregivers could not understand her speech. She exhibited frequent fits of "crying and yelling."

Her readings noted the paralysis and nervous system dysfunction. To address these conditions, the readings recommended electrotherapy and suggestive therapeutics:

Q. Is it possible to restore the cellular structure of this brain or to bring about compensatory action whereby the mind may again function perfectly in this body?

A. As indicated, if there is the ability for sufficient of the properties to be absorbed through the vibratory forces of the Gold impulse, and the suggestions for creative activities in the system are kept, it may be done. (1553-5)

There were also frequent recommendations pertaining to diet, massage, hydrotherapy, and laxatives. These were all commonly prescribed therapies in the readings and we will address them in the next chapter.

Fortunately in this case, abundant correspondence was exchanged which provides valuable insights into the progress of Mrs. [1553]. A few excerpts are provided to convey the general direction of treatment and therapeutic outcome:

May 23, 1939:

Mrs. [1553] seems to, at times, gain in strength and have a clear mental coordination—less emotional—less crying—yes, much less.

Her inability to speak articulately, except a very few understandable words, of course makes it difficult to know her feelings and her thoughts—but generally—there is improvement—great improvement as compared to a year ago when the first readings were had—you see, she started back from very close to "zero."

July 5, 1939:

Mother is certainly improving mentally—coordination. Now she asks to be read to—much of the time—but seems to be losing strength—vitality—seems languid.

September 10, 1939:

We feel mother is better, she now enjoys being read to very much, but constipation seems to be a big problem as it has always been.

December 19, 1939:

When I think of last Christmas time and then see how much better Mrs. [1553] is today it hardly seems possible, but it does make me so very thankful . . .

The extensive group of readings given for [1553] is exemplary in its depth and scope (a total of twenty-six readings were given). Virtually every issue which may arise in the treatment of dementia is addressed in this series.

While there was apparently significant progress made over a period of about 56 months, the condition was not cured. The question of additional progress was raised in reading 1553-26:

> Q. How much progress can we expect if we follow instruction?
> A. We may find fifty to seventy-five to ninety percent advance in the body becoming more normal again.

We do not know how much further progress, if any, was made in this case—there is insufficient follow-up data to allow a full evaluation.

In reading 1553-26 the question of diagnosis was also raised:

> Q. What would be the proper diagnosis of this case?
> A. As we find, in the present it is a complication arising from the old conditions caused first by the breaking of cellular forces, producing spasmodic conditions, then plastic conditions in portions of the body, and partial paresis [paralysis] to the nerve forces and to brain centers . . .

It is not clear whether the "breaking of cellular forces" referred to a stroke or some other acute illness. Paresis usually refers to a "partial or incomplete paralysis" *(Tabor's Cyclopedic Medical Dictionary)*. However, it can also refer to *dementia paralytica* (general paresis of the insane). This form of dementia is caused by syphilis and produces typical dementia symptoms including memory deficits, delusional thoughts, and depression.

The Case of [5204]

Mrs. [5204] was 51 years old when her husband wrote to Edgar Cayce requesting help for his wife:

> A personal friend of mine has recommended you to me as

one who may be able to tell me what is wrong with my wife. For 4 years now, my wife seems to have been losing her memory. She is unable to utter very many coherent sentences, and yet, she seems to understand what is being said to her. We have had her before innumerable doctors, and their diagnosis of her case has varied. We have been married 25 years and we have had a very happy home life, although the last 4 years have been very trying. She has forgotten how to do her housework and seems unable to cook a meal, although she always cooked our meals before. She has forgotten how to light the gas in the range, and we are fearful that something may happen to her. We no longer permit her to cook or attempt to cook. For a while, we thought that she was going through her menopause and this was causing the disturbance; but the doctors tell us that she has passed that stage . . . I am turning to you as a last resort . . . My wife is a very well-educated woman. She is kindly and sweet in disposition, and she went through college with honors, obtained Phi Beta Kappa honors, and was also a teacher of English in high school for a while. I have read Mr. Sugrue's book about you, and it has given me hope that I may still be able to save the life of a very sweet woman . . .

A subsequent letter written prior to her reading provided additional information which was addressed in her reading:

I am answering for my wife, because she does not feel well enough to do her own writing. She is anxious to know whether a blow on the head, caused by the falling of a flag-staff, has caused a tumor which makes her forget in the middle of a sentence when she attempts to converse. Or, also, if there is such a thing as the atrophying of the brain which may cause loss of memory; or whether her present period of forgetfulness is caused by menopausal period . . .

Edgar Cayce provided a reading for the woman on June 8, 1944:

As we find, there have been outside influences which have produced a real nervous shock to the system in such a nature that the reflexes from the cerebrospinal centers, and the cerebrospinal center itself, have received a condition which prevents their coordination.

These, as we find, reflect from clots which have formed on the capsule of the brain itself. They are not as tumors, rather as clots.

As we find, these may be removed by absorption or by operative measures. While it would require much longer for this to be done by absorption, it would be much more in accord with the insuring of longer experience in the earth . . . (5204-1)

The reading went on to recommend electrotherapy utilizing gold solution and spinal massage to induce "absorption" of the "clots." A positive prognosis was given provided the treatments were applied consistently:

These [treatments], if they are kept regularly, prayerfully, we may bring back memory, bring back coordination between cerebrospinal and sympathetic and the reflexes to the sensory system.

Given her history of brain insult (as documented in her husband's letters) and the connection between brain injury and dementia (see Chapter One), one wonders if the "outside influences" and "shock to the system" noted in her reading might have been caused by her being hit on her head by a falling flag-staff. Interestingly, an autopsy of her brain following her death in 1949 indicated that her condition was Alzheimer's dementia.

The suggestions in the reading were never followed completely. The family waited for one year after the reading was given to attempt applying the recommendations. The physician who was recommended by A.R.E. secretary Gladys Davis was never contacted.

Mrs. [5204]'s condition continued to deteriorate and was complicated by seizures. The correspondence does not indicate whether there was any correlation between the attempt at applying the recommendations and the seizures. At any rate, she was institutionalized in a private hospital and eventually was transferred to a state facility where she lived until her death.

This is the only documented case of Alzheimer's dementia in the Cayce readings. There are very likely numerous cases which would fit current diagnostic criteria. However, it is impossible to say with certainty since brain autopsies were seldom performed in such cases.

From a strictly statistical point of view, it is highly probable that several of the cases which we will discuss were Alzheimer's. The readings were given for thousands of individuals, many of whom were within the high risk area of the life span.

Even today, the only definitive means of identifying Alzheimer's dementia is by biopsy or autopsy. Unfortunately, [5204]'s case was the only one in the readings which was documented by this means.

The Case of [5299]

Mrs. [5299] was 57 years old when her daughter first wrote to Edgar Cayce requesting a reading for her mother. The excerpts which follow clearly indicate the seriousness of the situation:

> My mother just came home from Medical Center after being there 10 days for observation. Her case was called a rare brain disease and, as far as is known, there is no cure. She is losing the power of speech and has already lost the power to write, tell time or do any of the actions such as lacing shoes, etc. The doctors explained to me that between her brain and scalp there is only an air space and her brain cells are drying up one by one ... According to Medical Center this case of hers is not a form of insanity, as what little brain she has functions, but it is so pitiful ...
>
> Her diagnosis is Presenile Sclerosis, which is premature old age, along with hardening of the arteries and the part of her brain which controls the power of speech is affected. She is now getting pains in her head and we have no idea how long she will last. Her age is as of a woman in her eighties.

Her reading indicated a karmic and physical basis for her condition:

> As we find, here are disturbances which may not be other than materially aided. These are the results of karmic conditions for the body, as well as those about the body. We may help, yes.
>
> While there are the disturbances which are causing premature senile conditions, or the withering away of the control of mental reflexes, there should be care and loving kindness, gentleness and patience administered to the body. These will not only bring a greater attempt for the reactions but will bring

the greater ability for the soul-entity's development.

It would be well at times, as there are those bridges in the associations between the sympathetic and the cerebrospinal nerve forces, to be careful that the body does not injure itself or others; but do not put the body away, unless there becomes more of that which would be, or cause it to be, dangerous for others. (5299-1)

The treatment recommendations were typical for such cases—the use of the wet cell battery carrying a gold solution. This was to be followed by a thorough spinal massage.

A question posed near the end of her reading indicated that her symptoms were episodic—that is, she could function almost normally for short periods:

Q. In her present condition does she know what is going on around her, does she understand when spoken to or is it just certain times that her brain is completely normal?

A. Only at very small intervals. But we will find much improvement and a quieter reaction with the use of the Appliance and the massage. (5299-1)

Thus a cure was not promised, only "improvement and a quieter reaction." A request for a follow-up report was sent to her daughter. The letter was returned marked, "MOVED—LEFT NO ADDRESS." Thus, we do not know the outcome in this case.

The Case of Mrs. [3303]

We are not provided the age of Mrs. [3303]—only that she was over 50 years of age. A letter from her husband provided a medical diagnosis and a description of the primary symptom of her disorder—impaired memory:

She has not been told that she has cerebral arteriosclerosis, and seems to think she is all right—or at least near so—therefore she is a peculiarly hard case to deal with for doctors and myself. She was a brilliant professional pianist 35 years ago . . . but her memory had begun leaving her 10 years ago . . .

Edgar Cayce provided a reading for her which noted glandular dyfunctions and pressures along the spine as key causes of the disease:

> As we find, there are disturbing conditions with this body. These have at times been called varied names, owing to the age or the advanced stages of same. But the condition here arises from pressures that exist in relation to those changes in the glandular activity of the body . . .
>
> Thus the body becomes forgetful, absent-minded, unable to recall. There is not the reflex in the white and grey matter [of the nervous systems]. Thus these would eventually cause senility to the body, unless there are measures taken to supply new energies . . .
>
> Do these [treatments] and we will find much bettered conditions for this body; not only a retarding of this disintegration in nerve and blood supply but a replenishing and a building back to better conditions for this body. (3303-1)

The treatment recommendations were standard for such cases: spinal manipulations and massage, electrotherapy with gold, basic dietary suggestions, and exercise outdoors in the open.

This case is interesting since glandular dysfunction has been linked to Alzheimer's dementia (see Chapter One). Because the diagnostic system of that era did not recognize Alzheimer's dementia as a discreet pathological entity, but included cases of presenile dementia within the category of arteriosclerosis, this may have been a case of which would fit modern diagnostic criteria for Alzheimer's.

Cayce's acknowledgment that "These have at times been called varied names, owing to the age or the advanced stages of same" appears to recognize the diagnostic ambiguity of the disorder. He may have been referring to the distinction between presenile and senile dementia ("owing to the age or the advanced stages of same").

The Question of Senility

As we noted in Chapter One, until recently the term senility was commonly used synonymously with Alzheimer's dementia. Hence it is difficult to apply current diagnostic criteria to the conditions represented in the readings because at that time senility was generally viewed as a normal part of the aging process. Thus cases of dementia (and particularly Alzheimer's dementia) may not have been recognized as such. Furthermore, as just cited in the previous case study, this ambiguity extends to cases of arteriosclerosis. "Hardening of the arteries" and the resultant brain damage was viewed as the primary cause of Alzheimer's dementia. Therefore, in considering the cases in the readings, we can sometimes glean valuable information about the causes and treatment of dementia from readings classified as senility and arteriosclerosis.

For example, consider the case of [3631], a 72-year-old woman suffering from "mental lapses and melancholia [depression] during which periods she seems to turn on those she loves the best . . . "

Her reading acknowledged the seriousness of her condition:

> Here we find it is almost too late to undertake to keep this entity in this particular experience.
>
> As we find, disturbances here are those contingent with senility, and thus there is a wasting away of the impulses or the active forces within the nerve cells themselves—those reflexes that would attempt to occur in the brain . . . as memory, activity of the salivary glands, activity of the bladder.
>
> As we find, help is possible, but it will depend upon how consistently and persistently there would be the applications made that may renew nerve tissue and give life itself in the body-reaction. (3631-1)

In this selection, the phrase "wasting away of the impulses or the active forces within the nerve cells themselves" is suggestive of an organic degeneration within the brain.

The description of pathology within the brain of Mr. [3701] is even more explicit:

> These have to do primarily with senility; that is, impulse in the gray matter in nerve force is lacking. Thus gradually, unless measures are taken, there must come the softening of the brain cells so that the reflexes will gradually become less and less active for the flow of blood as well as impulse in the circulation through the central portion of brain . . . (3701-1)

Note the reference to "softening of the brain," a phrase often used in cases of dementia. Senility was also associated with softening of brain tissue in the case of [5309], a 60-year-old male:

Yes, here conditions are rather serious. From the injuries which have been received, there are the tendencies, from the jars to the body and the brain, for the softening or lack of virile energy being replenished; or senility. Thus tendencies for the lapses into a coma or semi-coma. (5309-1)

It would appear that in these cases the readings were using the term senility as it was commonly used during that era—as synonymous with an organic brain disorder manifesting as dementia. The readings noted that senility was usually age related, with senior citizens being more vulnerable. However, as we have noted and will reemphasize in the next chapter, Cayce also recognized the condition of "premature senility" (apparently in reference to the older classification of Alzheimer's disease, that is "presenile dementia").

Dementia Praecox

In addition to cases of senility, I would also recommend a consideration of cases of dementia praecox for those persons who are contemplating applying the Cayce suggestions. In the late nineteenth and early twentieth century, dementia praecox was the diagnostic category applied to persons suffering from chronic mental illness believed to be caused by brain disease. The term literally refers to an extremely early (precocious) form of dementia which is now included in the group of illnesses called schizophrenia. Whereas today the dementias are usually associated with the elderly, the symptoms of dementia praecox typically arose while individuals were in their late teens and early twenties.

It is not necessary for us to go deeply into this subject here and I only mention it for those individuals truly interested in understanding the readings' view of the dementias. I have written a treatment manual on schizophrenia which provides extensive documentation and a detailed consideration of the subject (see the Appendix for further information).

The primary value of this related material is in its application. The treatment suggestions for all the dementias were very similar. Since there was an abundance of readings on dementia praecox with explicit descriptions of therapeutic principles and techniques, this information represents an important source of supplemental data on the treatment of dementia in the elderly.

Cautious Optimism

It is crucial that readers recognize the difficulties involved in treating serious disorders such as the dementias. This book does not, in any way, suggest that Cayce's approach is "fool-proof" or easy to apply. To the contrary, Cayce often remarked that the suggestions provided in the readings would have to be carried out patiently and persistently if progress was to be achieved. He would then go on to say that if the persons administering the treatments were not dedicated to the healing process and willing to invest the resources necessary to follow the suggestions, it would be best that they not begin at all. However, for those willing to follow the suggestions in the readings, hope was provided.

The most unfortunate aspect of the Cayce readings in this area is the lack of application of the suggestions. For a variety of reasons (often of a financial nature; many of the readings were given during the "great depression"). Family members could not afford the recommended therapies. These cases were often chronic—the individuals involved came to Edgar Cayce as a last resort after years of failed treatment from numerous doctors and hospitals. Cayce's insistence that recovery would require patient and persistent treatment for a minimum of several months was apparently too much to ask of people discouraged by years of suffering.

In the few cases where there was consistent application of the suggestions provided in the readings, positive results were often produced. The previously discussed case of Mrs. [1553] is exemplary in this regard.

A letter from Edgar Cayce dated April 9, 1942, effectively conveys the cautious optimism with which he approached such cases:

> Am in hopes you have found the information for Miss [2721] of interest. Of course I realize what it means to raise false hopes in the minds of others. I realize anything I may say would appear as if I were blowing my own horn, but please know I realize too that it is not of myself the work is done, but only as the Spirit of Truth may work in or through me. We have had several cases of this nature that seemed hopeless, where seeming miracles have happened. There have been a few people sent to the Macon hospital [Still-Hildreth Osteopathic Sanatorium], so the work there will not be entirely new to them. Do hope you will write them and if it is possible or practical, do hope

you will give it a try. Have had many where the condition was not such as real help might be given, but where help has been promised [by the readings] through a certain mode of treatment, or by certain places or individuals, when this was done the help promised has come. Am sure, of the many thousands of readings that have been given, this has been true in practically every case. Many have, of course, been persuaded that the suggestions were all wrong and that the help suggested could not come from such a treatment, but where tried, whatever amount of help was offered has come. We will be glad to try and help anywhere along the line with checkup readings from time to time.

Do hope we may be the means of help, and may HIS blessings, His Peace come to you.

The reference to the Still-Hildreth Osteopathic Sanatorium was significant in this case. On numerous occasions, Cayce foresaw that the requirements for effective treatment would exceed the resources of the family as caregivers. Often in cases of dementia (such as dementia praecox), he would make a referral to Still-Hildreth. This institution utilized many of the therapeutic principles and techniques commonly advised in the readings.

This is relevant because many persons currently suffering from dementia are in nursing homes. For any approach to have a widespread impact upon the treatment of dementia, it would have to be integrated into existing institutional facilities. Therefore, it is worth noting that the principles advocated in Cayce's readings are applicable to an institutional setting. We will come back to this point in Chapter Six.

Summary

This chapter has explored an alternative perspective of the dementias. While acknowledging the severe brain pathology present in these disorders, the Cayce material goes further to emphasize the importance of the whole body (especially the peripheral nervous systems). Coordination between the central and autonomic nervous systems was specifically noted in the readings as being of great consequence.

However, Cayce's perspective goes beyond a mere biological analysis of pathology. The term holism was presented in this chapter to encompass the expansiveness of Cayce's perspective. All the aspects of the self are important—body, mind, and spirit. This emphasis on holism will become more prominent in the following chapters which focus on curative and preventative measures.

We reviewed several case studies from the Cayce material to get a firsthand look at his viewpoint. A variety of types of dementia were represented including a case of Alzheimer's disease. Since Alzheimer's dementia was not recognized as a formal diagnostic category during Cayce's lifetime, it is very likely that numerous other individuals received readings addressing this illness. However, they would likely have been diagnosed as "senility" or cardiovascular disease. Some examples of each were also presented to illustrate the similarities to present criteria for Alzheimer's dementia.

Finally, the theme of cautious optimism was introduced and balanced by the recognition of the difficulties involved in treating the devastating group of illnesses known as the dementias. The therapeutic approach underlying this hopeful perspective will be presented in the chapters which follow.

3

Therapeutic Options

◆

CONTEMPORARY APPROACHES TO the treatment of dementia begin with assessment. It is important to obtain an accurate diagnosis to insure that treatable dementias are identified and addressed. If a treatable dementia is diagnosed, specific therapeutic interventions can be attempted to address the specific cause. For instance, if the dementia is caused by a thyroid dysfunction, then a medication might be prescribed to correct the glandular imbalance.

In the case of Alzheimer's and other irreversible dementias, treatment is less specific and usually involves:

- general health maintenance measures (for example, improved nutrition, regular exercise, daily grooming, massage, etc.)
- behavioral interventions such as making lists, posting signs, and using alarm clocks to augment the failing memory and intellectual abilities of afflicted person
- medications to relieve/suppress mental symptoms such as anxiety, paranoia, and depression
- information and support to family members and friends so

that they can better cope with the symptoms of the disease

All of the above are *nonspecific* interventions aimed at making the best of a difficult situation. *Nonspecific* simply means that these interventions are applicable to a wide variety of disorders in addition to the dementias. In other words, they are not specifically directed at the cause of the dementia.

On the other hand, many *specific* treatments have been advocated for the irreversible dementias—particularly Alzheimer's dementia. These curative or "magic bullet" measures are sometimes attempted under the guise of research. Usually this amounts to giving some form of medication aimed at halting the deterioration or possibly even restoring a degree of functioning. The idea is to determine precisely what is causing the dementia and design a medication which will zero in on the problem at a neurobiological level.

Unfortunately, there are no generally acknowledged curative treatments currently available for Alzheimer's dementia. From time to time, researchers will declare a breakthrough such as a new medication only to find that further research fails to confirm the early claims of effectiveness.

Because there is undoubtedly a strong biological pathology associated with this dementia, research is likely to eventually produce more effective medications which will have widespread application. However, if such therapeutic breakthroughs follow the pattern set by the drugs used to treat the major mental illnesses, some problems will probably still remain. For example, these drugs tend to entail adverse side effects and variability of response (individuals may respond in varying degrees and some persons may not respond at all).

An Alternative Approach Based on the Cayce Readings

The Cayce readings actually proposed curative treatments for what we now call "reversible" and "irreversible" dementias. If the dementia had a specific cause which could be addressed, the readings would typically prescribe a therapy directed at the cause. If brain deterioration had advanced to a significant degree, the treatment plan would usually include the basic curative therapies used to treat "irreversible" dementia.

Interestingly, these curative treatments were also relatively nonspecific. In other words, the same basic treatments were recommended for the full spectrum of the dementias. Furthermore, these treatments were deemed appropriate for a wide range of disorders involving neurological impairment.

The foundation of Cayce's approach is the principle of self-healing. This refers to the body's innate tendency to heal itself. Thus, there is less emphasis on *specificity* because the body is doing the healing. Sometimes the body may require extensive assistance—yet the principle holds true. The important thing is that the treatments assist the body without getting in the way of natural healing processes.

Specificity does enter into therapy. However, it is found most often at the level of the individual rather than at the level of category of disease. In other words, the goal is to combine the basic treatments and fine tune the various techniques to suit the needs of each individual case regardless of whether the medical diagnosis is Alzheimer's dementia or some other neurological disorder.

"Building a New Brain"

Insofar as the readings on dementia are concerned, the focal point of self-healing is the reconstruction of the nervous system and particularly the brain. The use of "vibratory metals" (such as gold and silver) in conjunction with various forms of electrotherapy constitute the cornerstone of this approach:

> The PRINCIPLE [of using electrotherapy with gold or silver] being that these change the vibratory forces as they add to or take from impulses within the system, from which those of the sensory [nervous] system, or senses, react in the brain itself, and which takes place much as has been given with gold and silver in their varied conditions as may be applied to the system. We will find that impulse, whether as to that of senility when produced from age alone or whether senility as produced by conditions produced in the brain itself; for WITH the proper manipulations to PRODUCE coordination WITH drainage in the system, as may be given through manipulation osteopathically, or neuropathically given to the system under various stages, may create for a body almost a new brain, will the patience, the suggestion, the activities in the system BE carried out according to the conditions as necessary to be met. (1800-16)

Note the therapies mentioned in this excerpt: electrotherapy with gold and silver, osteopathic or neuropathic manipulations to produce "coordination WITH drainage in the system," patience, suggestion, and activities in the system (such as diet and medication). We will be addressing each of these interventions in this and subsequent chapters.

Also note the reference to "senility when produced from age alone or whether senility as produced by conditions produced in the brain itself." Keep in mind that dementias such as Alzheimer's disease were widely regarded as a form of senility during Cayce's era. In this reading, Cayce may have been acknowledging the prevalent diagnostic thinking which made a distinction between senile dementia ("senility . . . produced from age alone") and presenile dementia ("produced by conditions . . . in the brain itself"). He seemed to be saying that it did not matter how the disorder was classified, the treatment would be the same. Incidentally, this is essentially the same viewpoint which modern medical science has adopted toward Alzheimer's dementia several decades later. If you are confused over the distinction between senile and presenile dementia, you may wish to review the discussion in Chapter One which summarizes the history of classification of Alzheimer's dementia.

The assertion that one could "create for a body almost a new brain" is revolutionary in its implications and would undoubtedly be contested by current medical authorities. The readings acknowledged the incredulity which such an assertion would arouse:

> . . . there needs to be the character of application that would not only tear down the scar tissue made but replenish or rebuild the nerve tissue itself in [the] brain . . .
> This may be considered impossible, by some pathologists, or neurologists, or even some anatomists. Yet such has been done, and it may be done, in some instances . . .
> Now, the influences needed here are Gold, Silver and Camphor; Gold to the gray matter in nerve tissue itself; Silver in the cord of the white matter—that is the principal element or force or influence; Camphor as a healing agent—or that works with, or between, the two elements (in a vibratory force). (3071-1)

This excerpt was taken from a reading given for a 14-year-old boy suffering from cerebral palsy. Hence, the assertion that nerve tissue could be "rebuilt" was made on numerous occasions for a wide spectrum of neurological disorders, including the dementias.

It is important that we understand exactly what the readings meant by the expression "build a new brain." The intention was not that new nerve cells would necessarily be created. Rather, it was simply that the existing cells, which had atrophied or degenerated, were to be nourished and stimulated into a functional condition. It was a difficult process requiring time and patience on the part of the caregivers.

While electrotherapy with vibratory metals was essential for the rebuilding of nerve tissue, several other therapies play key roles in the healing process. As mentioned in the excerpt from reading 1800-16, spinal manipulations and massage were crucial ingredients. These therapies were directed at the major nerve plexus and ganglia throughout the system and especially along the spinal column. The purpose of manipulations was twofold: "to PRODUCE [1] coordination WITH [2] drainage in the system."

Do you recall the statement in Chapter Two emphasizing the importance of coordination between the cerebrospinal and sympathetic nervous systems in the treatment of dementia? (See reading excerpt 5475-1.) Establishing this coordination was a primary goal of the spinal manipulations and massage. The techniques of massage and adjustments involved were a hallmark of the physical therapies practiced by the osteopathic and neuropathic physicians of that era.

While the spinal manipulations were typically given by the professional during bi-weekly trips at the office, the spinal massage was often given by the family caregiver at home immediately following the electrotherapy. Reading 1553-5 explicitly described the therapeutic effects provided by the spinal massage:

Q. What will this Vibratory Gold Solution and massage treatment accomplish?

A. It SHOULD accomplish that as we have indicated. As to what, it will depend upon the purpose and manner with which the treatments are administered. The massage only assists the impulse for activity from the nerve centers and ganglia to be directed in the activities of the functioning portions of the system that are controlled by certain reflexes or certain impulses created in same. Just as in that where there may be a clogged line or a dammed stream. If there are particles removed, it allows the greater flow of activity. And these impulses for mental and physical reaction are necessary for the body to coordinate properly. Hence the massage should assist in the impulses being carried from assimilated forces to the activities of the mental, the physical and the spiritual self. (1553-5)

Thus, coordination was increased by "unclogging" the nerve plexus and ganglia thereby allowing the impulses to pass freely to the organs of the system. The pattern of spinal massage and manipulation was often specified in the readings along with a mixture of oils to be rubbed into the body to "feed," as it were, the nerve tissue. Here is a brief selection which illustrates the type of massage frequently recommended:

These [massages] should be a gentle, circular motion along each side of the cerebrospinal centers—that is, along the side of the spine, or the sympathetic nerve system, circular motion downward; across especially the abdominal, through the groin and down the limb—circular motion always—these areas especially. (1553-16)

The second major objective of the manipulations and massage was to set up drainages within the system. This means that the eliminative systems were to be engaged to increase the body's ability to remove wastes, particularly the byproducts of metabolism. Improving and maintaining good eliminations was emphasized because the electrotherapy with the vibratory metals was intended to stimulate the glandular activity necessary for rebuilding the nervous systems. The rebuilding process would necessarily produce a great deal of waste that would need to be evacuated from the diseased tissue. The manipulations were to stimulate the major plexus which connect to the organs of elimination throughout the system. Hence:

The manipulations, or the points of contact, as we find may aid the better eliminations a great deal by the paralleling of either side along the area in the 6th to the 9th dorsal with those centers from which the sphincter muscular forces in the lumbar and sacral receive their impulse. These, with the other suggested applications in adjustments, would be well. (1553-17)

Hydrotherapy, laxatives, and dietary recommendations were also frequently combined with the manipulations to enhance eliminations. Hydrotherapy often included enemas or colonics to cleanse the lower bowel.

According to the readings, setting up proper eliminations is a bit of a balancing act. Eliminations must be balanced for best results:

> Q. Is the elimination now enough for this body?
> A. At times, yes. At others, not sufficient. For remember, most of the poisons of the body must be through the drainages or drosses through the alimentary canal; especially for one of this temperament and this age. Do not increase the eliminations so as to be a drain upon the system, but do not allow the low or slow activity to reproduce poisons that become as toxic conditions gradually in the body. (1553-22)

Naturally, the laxatives which were recommended were mild. The readings often preferred to alternate between mineral and vegetable laxatives so the eliminating systems would not become totally dependent upon outside forces and thereby lose the ability to function normally. Diet was also suggested to improve eliminations. We will discuss dietary recommendations in a later section.

So, with improved coordination between the nervous systems and better eliminations established to clean up the internal environment, the way would be prepared for the use of the vibratory metals to stimulate nerve repair. Let's look more closely at how this vibratory healing might actually be accomplished.

How Do Vibratory Metals Work?

Keep in mind that the form of electrotherapy recommended by the readings in most cases of dementia was extremely mild. The most frequently suggested appliance was the Wet Cell, a simple chemical battery which delivers a very minute direct current. A glass jar containing the desired solution was generally incorporated into the electrical circuit before attachment to the body.

Most people feel little or no physical sensation during this form of electrotherapy. In fact it is so extremely mild that one wonders how it could possibly produce such remarkable results as nerve tissue regeneration.

The answer is we simply don't know precisely how it could work. Modern technology and theories are just beginning to explore the role of "subtle energies" in the human body.

Catering to my own curiosity in this matter, I have developed a theory of how "vibratory" substances could work. Keep in mind it is only a model to help me understand this ambiguous subject. And yet, it might be helpful to others, so I will pass it along for what it is worth.

Recognize that the body is an enormously complex chemical factory. We ingest food, inhale air, and eliminate wastes at an incredible rate. All these biological processes entail complicated chemical reactions and energy transformations.

Imagine that the various chemicals in our body serve as messengers bearing information to the organs of the body. The information may be simple or complex depending upon its function. However, its essential purpose can be described simply. For example, the information could function like a purchase order in a business transaction. It might request that a certain organ release into the blood supply a particular substance that the organ either has in store or can produce on command. The various messengers can thus regulate the kind and amount of various secretions in the body. Up to this point, medical science has fairly well documented the information exchange within the molecular structure of our bodies—even down to the DNA which is the hereditary template governing the processing and distribution of chemical information.

While recognizing these basic biochemical processes, the Cayce readings go further into the workings of the body and describe vibratory patterns of assimilation and distribution. This aspect of human physiology is at the cutting edge of biological theory and research. A group of scientists and health care practitioners have formed an organization to study the nature of this phenomenon and to empirically document its existence through controlled studies. This group has designated itself the International Society for the Study of Subtle Energies and Energy Medicine (ISSSEEM). Readers desiring further information about the vibratory or subtle energy dimension of the body may wish to contact this organization and obtain further information about this phenomenon (see the Appendix).

Here is a brief explanation that helps me to understand what the readings mean when they speak of vibratory energies. Keep in mind that this is only a theory among many theories and is presented to help you to get a foothold on the concept of vibratory phenomenon.

We are all constantly deluged by various kinds of information. This information can take many forms, some of which we process through our five physical senses. We hear, see, smell, feel, and on occasion even taste our immediate environment. It is well understood by scientists that we are conscious of only a very small amount of the information which engulfs us. Some of this information is quite subtle.

Take for example the abundant information contained in starlight. Unless we are astronomers, we hardly take notice of our celestial neighbors. With the high levels of environmental pollution, we may even have trouble seeing them on a cloudless night. Yet through a sophisticated process of spectral-analysis, scientists can determine the chemical makeup and physical properties of stars which produced the light billions of miles away and many years ago. In fact, the stars themselves may even no longer exist. And yet the vibratory pattern, a sort of energy signature of their identity, has traveled through space all this time. The light acts as a messenger for a specific kind of information about the elemental composition of the star. With the right equipment and technical expertise, we can interpret this subtle energy message.

Perhaps a similar process occurs in the human body. Perhaps part of the digestive process serves to break down substances into their elemental components. After processing by the visceral organs, the vibrational signature of these substances are carried via the basic biochemical energy transfers which maintain the body. So that, just like the starlight, the end result is a transfer of information via energy.

I used the example of starlight because it is such a faint carrier of the star's vibratory signature. I could have used more immediate and powerful examples such as the way voice patterns are carried along a telephone wire or TV signals are transferred via electromagnetic waves. Just as there are varying levels of energy patterns in our external environment, our bodies also probably utilize multiple energy systems. Some may even be more subtle than starlight and yet capable of carrying information.

That the human body could incorporate such intricate information systems into its physiology does not seem implausible to me. There is so much about the body that we do not presently understand, I think it is reasonable that we at least stay open to such possibilities.

The readings regard the reality of vibratory systems within the body as more than a possibility. In fact, these systems are mentioned frequently, especially in the context of the various therapies and how they work. For instance, the use of the Wet Cell Battery with gold or silver follows specific patterns which incorporate some of the major nerve plexus of the body. In most cases the attachments are to be placed over the umbilical plexus and the enlarged ganglia of the sympathetic nervous system. It is stated in the readings that these strategic nerve centers allow the vibratory influence to be transmitted to the glands of the system (especially the endocrine glands). According to the readings, these glands secrete hormones necessary for the proper functioning of the nervous systems.

Using the model which I have presented, we could consider the vibratory influence of substances such as gold and silver as a form of information provided to the glands signaling the need to produce a certain type of secretion. The type of rebuilding required determines the type of information that must be transmitted to the glands. For example, within the nervous system, there are two broad classes of tissue—the gray matter and the white matter. The recommendations in the readings took into consideration the type of tissue which required regeneration:

> Now, the influences needed here are Gold, Silver and Camphor; Gold to the gray matter in nerve tissue itself; Silver in the cord of the white matter . . . Camphor as a healing agent—or that works with, or between, the two elements (in a vibratory force) . . . (3071-1)

In most cases of dementia, it was the gold that was recommended. Presumably, the primary pathology was to the gray matter in nerve tissue.

As I stated before, this is just a possible explanation of a process which the readings describe as the body's vibratory energies. I only pass it along as a educational tool to help you to understand the therapeutic techniques which utilize vibratory substances.

Suggestive Therapeutics

Let us focus briefly on a powerful hypnotic technique for dealing with behavioral problems and facilitating the healing process. *Suggestive therapeutics* is the term applied to a form of natural hypnosis which the readings often recommended in cases of dementia. Because most persons are unfamiliar with the techniques for inducing a hypnotic trance, the readings advised that suggestions be provided *during* the physical treatments while the person was in a relaxed, receptive state of mind. Thus during the electrotherapy, massage, and manipulations the caregiver was directed to talk to the patient in a calm, firm voice; giving positive suggestions for physical, mental, and spiritual healing. The suggestions could also be directed towards undesirable behaviors or lack of cooperation. Here is an example of suggestive therapeutics from the [1553] series of readings:

> As to the suggestions that should be given—when there are the administrations of ANY of the influences for aid, whether the rubs or the packs or whatnot, the suggestions should be of a very positive nature, yet very gentle, and in a constructive way and manner; expressing hope always that there is a creating, through the hope, the expectancy for certain activities to the body that it desires to do—much in the manner as would be given to a child in its promptings for an aid to itself.
>
> And, let the suggestions be constructive in the spiritual sense, when the manipulations or adjustments are given, as well as when there are the periods of the rubs and other applications. These would be well in this manner, though each individual should construct same in his or her own words:
>
> "Let there be accomplished through the desires of this body, mentally and physically, that which will enable the body to give the better, the truer, the more real expression of its own self; as well as that in which the entity or body may influence itself in relationships to others for greater physical, mental and spiritual attitudes towards conditions."
>
> Then, let the desire of the body through ALL its activities in the present be of a spiritual nature . . .
>
> Q. Should suggestions be made by BOTH the Doctor and those taking care of her?
>
> A. Just as indicated, these should be made whenever any applications are made—whether for the rubs, the adjustments, or the packs. The BODY desires attention—but in a manner in which there are, as indicated, the suggestions that it is to become not so reliant upon others, but so—because of the very nature of the applications—that it may do more and more for itself. Whenever there is the suggestion, it should be not as "There WON'T be," but "You WILL do so and so," see?
>
> Q. What can we do for the crying—nervousness and her refusing to drink?

A. This can only be met through the suggestions—for, as has been indicated, these periods come and go; and, as has been outlined heretofore, it is a lack of the coordinating between the cerebrospinal and sympathetic [nerve] impulses or reflexes. (1553-17)

The readings also frequently advised that bedtime be utilized as a period for suggestive therapeutics. During the first few minutes of sleep, a slumbering individual is in a hypnogogic state and is very open to suggestion. This form of suggestive therapeutics is sometimes referred to as pre-sleep suggestions. As with all forms of suggestive therapeutics, pre-sleep suggestions are made to the person's unconscious mind and should be positive and constructive in tone and content.

The Role of Diet

The readings generally recommended a balanced diet in cases of dementia. Foods which are easily assimilated were emphasized. If meats were to be taken, seafoods and fowl were suggested rather than pork and beef. Fruits and vegetables were recommended with an emphasis on vegetables grown above ground. Whole grain products such whole wheat bread were preferred. While dairy products of all kinds were generally acceptable in moderation, carbonated drinks were not.

Obviously, such a diet would tend to improve eliminations. In certain cases where the body was very weak, a blood and nerve building diet was recommended:

In the diets, as we find now—the vitamins that create a better blood and nerve activity are most desired. Then, let there be regular periods when liver or those foods of such natures would be given in proportions as the body may desire—broiled, not fried, and never hard—but the juices of same should always be given with same. Use steel cut oats, and especially the oyster plant, and also other vegetables that are of the same nature. These carry influences that are very necessary and beneficial, especially if cooked in their OWN juices (as in Patapar Paper) and seasoned to the taste. (1553-17)

The Edgar Cayce Foundation has produced an extremely helpful laminated one-page diet guide entitled *Diet Basics from the Edgar Cayce Readings.* This handy chart can be posted in the kitchen area for easy reference. There are numerous other resources available which explain the readings' approach to diet and nutrition and we need not go deeply into this subject here (see the Appendix).

The Spiritual Dimension of Therapy

The readings maintain a strong spiritual emphasis in cases of dementia. Accordingly, it is the patience, persistence, gentleness, and kindness with which the therapies are given which makes healing possible. These qualities are sometimes referred to as "fruits of the spirit." Hence it is the spirituality of the caregivers which makes treatment more than a technical procedure. Cayce insisted that the treatments not be given merely as rote, as something to be gotten through with as quickly as possible. From the perspective of the readings, such an attitude impoverishes treatment of any kind.

The readings also emphasize the opportunity for personal growth on the part of the caregivers. In certain cases, loving treatment was even characterized as a karmic obligation on the part of close relatives. We will further consider some of these spiritual issues of treatment in the next chapter when we examine the meaning of healing.

Summary

Some of the "reversible" dementias can be treated effectively if they are accurately diagnosed and treated early. However, there exists no recognized curative treatment for Alzheimer's dementia. Current therapeutic approaches emphasize general health maintenance and behavioral management to minimize the undesirable symptoms of the disease.

The Cayce readings also stress the importance of general health maintenance and behavioral interventions as a means of lessening the impact of these disorders. The readings digress from the modern medical model by stressing the importance of allowing the body to heal itself. There is a strong emphasis on the concept that all healing is spiritual in nature and that healing comes from within, regardless of the form of treatment which is used to stimulate the healing process.

"Natural" remedies play a major role in stimulating the body's capacity to heal itself. The readings insist that even the brain can be assisted in regeneration in certain cases by the use of vibratory medicines (such as gold and silver) and certain basic adjunct therapies.

To assist in summarizing the treatments commonly recommended in cases of dementia, I have put together an outline of basic therapies which were most often suggested:

1. Spinal manipulations to help coordinate the nervous systems and improve eliminations

2. Electrotherapy with gold (and in certain cases with silver and camphor)

3. Massage immediately following the electrotherapy (emphasis on the ganglia along the spine and the visceral organs of assimilation and elimination)

4. Suggestive therapeutics to constructively engage the healing powers of the mind and modify behavioral problems

5. Hydrotherapy to improve eliminations

6. Balanced diet of wholesome foods which are easily assimilated and eliminated (blood and nerve building diet in certain cases where the whole body is weak)

7. Spiritual attitude on the part of the caregivers

This book is not intended to be a treatment manual—rather, it is simply an introduction to the therapeutic principles and techniques most commonly recommended in the readings on dementia. For those persons wishing to apply this information, I have put together a treatment manual which addresses nervous system regeneration (*Principles & Techniques of Nerve Regeneration: Alzheimer's Disease and the Dementias;* see the Appendix). Naturally, anyone wishing to apply this approach should contact a qualified health care professional to assist in the various therapies discussed in this chapter.

4

The Meaning of Healing

◆

LIVING IN A materialistic culture, it is so easy to view disease as simply a physical disorder. Although attitudes towards health and illness are changing in this regard (we are becoming more aware of the psychological and social dimensions of illness), the usual response to disease is strongly biological. In short, we tend to rely heavily on drugs or other "physical" therapies to cure whatever ails us.

In the previous chapters we have paid considerable attention to the biological aspects of the dementias. We have looked at several possible causes and considered some alternative therapies for treating these disorders of the body.

To gain a full understanding of Edgar Cayce's perspective on this subject, we must now take a broader view. We must consider not only the whole body, but also include the interpersonal and transpersonal aspects of healing.

In Chapter Three we noted Edgar Cayce's emphasis on self-healing (all healing comes from within). Yet, as a rule, demented individuals cannot heal themselves to any great extent. The nature and seriousness of the illness usually block the healing process. For it is the physical interface of mind and spirit with the body that is disrupted in dementia. Particularly, the nervous systems are so adversely affected that healing from within is difficult, if not impossible. Cayce's oft-quoted observation that "mind is the builder" does not easily apply here. How can the mind serve in the interest of healing when it is the mind itself that is the problem. Mind cannot effectively operate through a degenerated nervous system.

Consequently, the help of other persons (other minds, if you will) who are willing to invest in the healing process is essential. In this chapter we will closely examine the role of caregivers in treating dementia.

As we shall see, this role involves more than just providing a series of treatments. The treatments do not heal. At best, they can only help the body to restore its natural capacity for self-healing.

Herein lies a major difficulty in treating degenerative disorders such as the dementias. Sometimes the response from within does not come. For a variety of reasons, not all of which are physical, the body may have lost its gift of healing. In other words, sometimes there are limits to physical healing, as we shall see later in this chapter.

The Context of Healing

Regardless of the illness, the readings consistently emphasized the importance of purposeful living. This was especially true in cases of severe and prolonged disability where the healing process could be long and arduous.

Often, when the stricken individual would ask questions pertaining to the length of time required for recovery or even if recovery were a possibility, the readings would respond with some basic question about the reason for desiring health. Why would you be healed? How would you live your life differently? Why are you alive? Why continue living?

These questions address an essential aspect of the healing process—the spiritual dimension. They involve the purpose, meaning, and value of life. Finding the answers to these basic questions requires soul searching. In a certain sense, all catastrophic illness addresses these questions at some level. During such distress, we are encouraged to tune in to the spiritual dimension; to pay close attention to our thoughts and feelings; to decide what our lives are about; to choose our future.

Such deep questions take on an added dimension in the context of an apparently irreversible degenerative illness. The sufferer may not even have the mental resources to understand these questions or respond in a coherent manner. In such cases, Cayce insisted that the load of responsibility falls on the caregivers to acknowledge the source of healing and the consequences of health.

This is where the spiritual qualities of the caregivers come into play. Through the application of the "fruits of the spirit," the sufferer may be awakened to the possibilities of living. Gentleness, kindness, patience, and persistence are powerful interventions which touch the spiritual essence of everyone, regardless of the state of health.

Talking (or writing) about spiritual application in healing is easy. Living it can be excruciatingly difficult. Reading 271-7 was given for a man suffering from dementia. The excerpt which follows effectively captures the daily frustration of caregivers attempting to follow Cayce's treatment plan:

> As to how the associates are to accomplish same [the treatments], it requires patience and persistence, and prayer, and understanding; and if these are not being accomplished they are untrue first to selves and to the duty and obligation that is about those who would direct the changes that are being made in the applications of those things that have started in the bringing about of the reactions in the body.
>
> Then, in making the applications for the conditions in the system, where the electrical forces are adding to the motivative forces of the body, these should be kept as near intact with that which has been given as possible. To be sure, fear of what will be the result is the basic principle that prevents the body from being docile; but, if the body were docile—then you'd know he was already an ass and would never be much else!
>
> But the conditions to be met are in that of patience, persistence, and reasoning with the body for the better improvement of its own abilities to meet the needs of the varied conditions that arise in the activities of the body itself. Not because "Your mammy wants it," not because "You've got to do it," but because "This will make for the better reactions in yourself!" For there are periods when the reactions are near normal.
>
> The periods then of what may be termed rationality, in rea-

soning, are longer; they may not be but a moment longer, but to this experience that may mean many years of sane rationalism, if those moments are taken advantage of. Ready for questions.

Q. What approach should Lu make to get [271] to take the [Wet Cell] battery . . .

A. This has just been given, as to how the approach is to be made; with patience, with persistence. Rather than losing patience and saying harsh words, walk away! Then, when self has gained control of self, just reason—and reason—and reason.

Q. When he absolutely refuses to have the battery, is it best to wait until the next night?

A. Best to wait if it's a hundred years; wait until you have succeeded in conquering self, and you will then be able to conquer the body and the mind! If it's a day, or a night, or a week, a month, a year, conquer self!

Q. Is there any way this fear in the body can be removed?

A. By the patience, persistence of suggestion to the body. Is there any way that to the mind of a child that has been burned, it can be taught there is a way to handle fire? This is gradually builded by the overcoming of fear, through the suggestions—patiently, persistently; patiently, persistently; prayerfully. (271-7)

So there is more involved in treating dementia than simply providing physical treatment and waiting for results. In the previous case, the caregivers are encouraged to awaken their own spirituality. In order to conquer the illness in this man's body, they had to first conquer their own impatience. They had to develop the impulse control that would prevent them from losing their temper. They had to acquire the faith that would enable them to take the bigger view; when even small gains were being made, to trust that their efforts were not wasted.

Another way of considering the role of spirituality in the healing process is to look closely at the attitude of the caregiver:

While, true, medicines, compounds, mechanical appliances, radiation, all have their place and are of the creative forces, yet the personality of arousing hope, of creating confidence, of bringing the awareness of faith into the consciousness of an individual is very necessary. (5083-2)

Make such applications more as not merely something to be gotten through with, but more as a part of entertainment to the body, as well as having the body enter into the treatments with more the air of expectancy. This should be the attitude on the part of each one making the applications. (1553-18)

Having a positive attitude while giving the treatments involves an element of faith—faith in service, trusting that the work that is done will bear fruit. The fruition may not be immediate or dramatic. In fact, in cases of dementia, positive results may require a substantial investment of time and effort before paying off:

If there are the conclusions that the treatment won't do any good (because the relief doesn't happen in the moment), then don't try it! (2575-2)

Q. Has the massage been given properly?
A. Very good. Just as we have indicated, be mindful in the massage that it doesn't become merely a period that "I must give him the treatment and be through with it," but that it will be accomplished if it will be applied in this way and manner. (448-2)

One of the most powerful incentives for caregivers to maintain a positive mental attitude is the recognition that "mind is the builder." According to Cayce and many other metaphysical sources, the thoughts and images we hold in our minds are real and will inevitably manifest in physical reality in some form. Our most intimate mental constructions are our own physical bodies. In a similar vein the biblical scriptures observe, "As a man thinketh in his heart, so he is."

Yet, how can mind be the builder when the mind is demented? If the nervous systems are degenerated to the point of affecting the way a person thinks, what can the mind build? When persons have lost much of the capacity to remember and may even be experiencing delusions and hallucinations, how can they be expected to utilize their minds in the healing process?

The answer is simply that it is the mind of the caregivers that must do the building. The beliefs and attitudes of those around the afflicted individual provide the mental programming that informs the body to heal itself. We have already considered one of the interpersonal techniques for such programming. In Chapter Four the concept of suggestive therapeutics was introduced and explained. In suggestive therapeutics, constructive information is spoken directly to the patient by the caregiver during the therapies and at bedtime.

However, the readings went beyond suggestive therapeutics in describing the influence of the caregiver's attitudes and beliefs. Cayce stated that the entire healing environment must be positive and constructive.

For example, consider the programming that a demented person might receive from many television shows portraying graphic violence. The readings explicitly describe how the sensory nervous system picks up such information from the environment and relays it to the brain and sympathetic nervous system for storage within the cellular structure. Presumably the physical treatments are to stimulate the brain and nervous systems of the body to rebuild and "reprogram" themselves. Thus, environmental cues automatically become part of the patient's mental being.

The technical term for the concept of environmental influence is "therapeutic milieu." Milieu simply means environment or surroundings. Thus, we are speaking here of providing a healing environment in all its aspects. Naturally, this would include clean facilities with sufficient stimulation to provide interesting and worthwhile interactions—and yet, not giving way to every wish and whim of the patient.

In this way the total environment acts in a suggestive way toward the patient. Arranging and maintaining a constructive environment is the responsibility of the caregivers. Therefore, the foundation of any therapeutic milieu is the attitudes and values of the caregivers. This leads us right back to treatment as a spiritual experience for all persons involved. The attitudes, beliefs, values, and behaviors of the caregivers lay the groundwork for personal growth and healing for everyone involved in the therapeutic process.

Regardless of the eventual outcome in strictly physical terms, this process does inevitably provide some degree of healing for the healer. The readings refer to this as soul growth.

All Healing Comes from Within

The medical model of healing, which underlies most contemporary therapeutic interventions, is largely based on the assumption that treatment produces healing. The Cayce readings prefer to em-

phasize that it is attunement within the body that produces healing—not the treatments. In other words, in certain cases the correct
treatment can be given and the body may simply not respond. In a
serious illness such as dementia, one must not simply provide treatment in a mechanical fashion (as if the treatment is all there is to it),
but seek to produce attunement within the inflicted individual.

The most obvious ramification of this principle is the problem of
reaction within individuals suffering from dementia. When there is
actual brain degeneration, the reaction of the body to treatment
may be difficult to maintain. In several cases, Cayce cautioned that
a "wait and see" attitude would be necessary because deterioration
was so advanced that a positive prognosis was problematic.
Caregivers were cautioned to follow the suggested treatment plan
and see if the body would respond. The spiritual dimension of the
applications was strongly emphasized in these cases. One can sense
Cayce's transpersonal perspective in these instances—the unconscious (or "soul forces") would have to be stimulated to regenerate
the physical body. Without such a response from the "divine within
self," recovery was impossible.

To emphasize the importance of the body's response to treatment
(that is, the response of the "divine within self"), I have assembled
several important excerpts from the readings to underscore this
limitation to healing:

> Q. May the body expect a complete cure? If so, how long will
> it be?
> A. This depends, naturally, upon the reactions and the man-
> ner in which the applications may be made—as to the re-
> sponses to and by the body. These, of course, are always
> questions—where body-building has to be accomplished. But
> if there is the change see, then the more hopefulness being
> held, the greater the change may be. (1310-1)

> Q. Would it be satisfactory to continue—
> A. [Interrupting] You see, it is not that there are just so many
> treatments to be given and they can all be gotten through with
> and that's all there is to it! NO application of ANY medicinal
> property or any mechanical adjustment, or any other influ-
> ence, is healing of itself! These applications merely help to at-
> tune, adjust, correlate the activities of the bodily functions to
> nature and natural sources!

All healing, thence is from life! Life is God! It is the adjusting of the forces that are manifested in the individual body.

These directions as we have indicated take these conditions into consideration. Then, there must be periods of reaction of the bodily forces, the bodily functionings, the bodily response to influences without and within; and then the necessary attuning again and again.

The BODY is a pattern, it is an ensample of all the forces of the universe itself.

If all the rain that is helpful for the production of any element came at once, would it be better? If all the sunshine came at once, would it be better? If all the joy, all the sadness in the life experience of an individual were poured out at once, would it be better?

It is the cooperation, the reaction, the response made BY the individual that is sought. Know that the soul-entity must find in the applications that response which attunes its abilities, its hopes, its desires, its purposes to that universal consciousness.

THAT is the healing—of any nature! (2153-6)

Here, then, we find the disturbances:

Pressures in the cerebrospinal areas that reflect to the ganglia along the centers in the cerebrospinal [nervous] system. While there has not been the response to some applications that have been made, these have been more in the nature of purely mechanical adjustments without consideration of the interchanging activity of body, mind and spiritual influences in the body.

KNOW—KNOW—there CAN be NO healing save from the awakening of the divine within self. This is not only true for this body but every individual entity. It is a fact that these influences or centers may be aroused by varied means, through which body, mind and soul function in the physical being. Thus the needs of these considerations for this body, particularly, in making administrations for beneficial results for this body! (2642-1)

Q. Can he be taught to dress, feed, and care for himself in other respects?

A. If there is any response, much may be accomplished through this. If there is no response, little—or none—can be accomplished. It will require patience and persistence. See? ... This, as is seen, must be builded within the mental being of the body. (5598-1)

These excerpts clearly acknowledge the role of the body in healing itself. Without the response from within, healing will not occur.

At this point, we have a bit of a dilemma for the caregivers in cases of dementia. If physical healing is not a certainty; if the body does not necessarily and automatically respond to therapy; how can one maintain an attitude of hopefulness and expectancy? How does one maintain faith in the face of such uncertainty?

The answer is simply that personal growth is a certainty if a spiritual emphasis in maintained. Rebuilding of the nervous system is not a certainty. A return to complete normalcy is not a certainty. The guarantee lies in the promise that the good work that is done is never in vain. Regardless of the degree of physical healing that is accomplished, all persons involved do grow at a deep level of being—at a soul level.

The concept of soul development for all concerned is inherent in the healing process and is explicitly stated in a reading given for a fifty-seven-year-old woman suffering from dementia:

As we find, here are disturbances which may not be other than materially aided. These are the results of karmic conditions for the body, as well as those about the body. We may help, yes.

While there are the disturbances which are causing premature senile conditions [presenile dementia], or the withering away of the control of mental reflexes, there should be care and loving kindness, gentleness and patience administered to the body. These will not only bring a greater attempt for the reactions but will bring the greater ability for the soul-entity's development. (5299-1)

This reading went on to recommend the full range of physical treatments commonly suggested in such cases (which have been documented in previous chapters).

The linkage of physical treatment with soul development is not implausible. In fact, consistent application of the various types of treatment recommendations in the readings will invariably lead to such growth. These therapies require that one apply spiritual principles on a daily basis. The necessity of applying spiritual qualities such as patience, persistence, gentleness, and kindness are built into the treatment plan, so to speak.

So while on the surface Cayce's approach has a strong physical or biological emphasis, be aware of its foundation in spiritual principles. The bottom line is: you cannot really use this approach without applying the "fruits of the spirit." Therefore, applying this approach with any degree of consistency will invariably lead to soul development for all involved.

The Limits of Physical Healing

Even in cases of dementia, where the physical degeneration had progressed to the point where the soul was not able to maintain a viable connection with the body, the readings insisted that the departed soul would benefit from the gentleness and kindnesses provided through the physical treatments.

For example, Ms. [5344] was only thirty-three years old when she suffered a nervous breakdown. About a year later she was given a reading which diagnosed her case as dementia and noted:

> There has already been departure of the soul, which only waits by here. We have the physical being but the control of same only needs the care, the attention, the greater love which may be shown in and under the circumstances, which will give the best conditions for this body. (5344-1)

Similarly, the caregivers of [586] were admonished to provide loving care to the physical shell which had been departed due to a weakening of the connections between body, mind, and spirit.

> For there has much that many would study in such a case departed from the surroundings of this body . . .
>
> The coordination has been severed between that which is of the physical-physical and the mental and spiritual activities as a unit.
>
> As we find, little may be added, save for the comfort of this body.
>
> While, through the concerted efforts of those that would in-

duce a regeneration of the body mentally, spiritually, there
might be brought to the body a more awareness of its condition, this—from here—we would not advise . . .
    Q. Is there any advice for those who would help this body?
    A. Let that be done in a manner as to keep as much of the
quiet and as free from physical pain as may be done. (586-1)

Obviously, there are limits to physical healing. In cases of severe
brain deterioration, Cayce usually left the question of whether to
undertake a regenerative regimen to the caregivers to decide. After
all, they were the ones who had to provide the treatments and/or
pay the bills. Whatever the ultimate decision regarding treatment,
loving care of the body was always emphasized.

Summary

In this chapter we have considered some of the mental and spiritual aspects of healing. We have looked at the importance of constructive mental attitudes on the part of caregivers. We have
recognized the necessity of the "fruits of the spirit" such as patience
and persistence. We have noted that all healing comes from within
and that the response of the body is essential for physical regeneration. Finally, we have cautioned that there are limits to physical
healing; especially when nervous system degeneration is so extreme
so as to prevent the soul from manifesting in a human body.
    Clearly, treating dementia involves more than simply hooking the
person up to an electrical appliance or giving a spinal massage.
While the various physical treatments are important, the deeper issue of the purpose of healing must be addressed. It is important to
analyze the purpose for undertaking a regimen of healing, particularly in cases of dementia where the burden of consistent treatment
is considerable. Naturally, we all want to alleviate the suffering of
other human beings. But precisely what are we expecting to achieve
by our efforts? Full physical healing and the restoration of functioning? Halting or slowing the deterioration so as to minimize the impact of the illness? Providing comfort and hope to a soul near the
end of an earthly existence?
    All of these goals are desirable and worthy of our efforts. Further-
more, from the perspective of the readings, these are all attainable
objectives in varying degrees (depending upon the quality of treatment and response of the body). However, it is important to keep in

mind that the healing process is about change. The aim is the trans-
formation of each person involved in the healing process. In this
chapter we have defined this transformative experience as soul development. Therein lies the meaning of healing.

5

Prevention

◆────────

PREVENTION HAS BECOME a hot topic in the current health care literature. While there has been a health-oriented magazine bearing that name for many years, it has only been recently that the health care crisis has pushed mainstream thinking in a preventative direction. Now, one may even find major hospitals offering health maintenance and preventative programs with increasing frequency.

The readings of Edgar Cayce were decades ahead of this preventative trend. They contain abundant suggestions for maintaining health through natural means. Some of the recommendations are *specific* (such as utilizing weekly peanut oil rubs to prevent arthritis or eating a couple of almonds each day to lessen the chances of developing cancer). Other recommendations are *nonspecific*. That is, the recommended regimen may be helpful in preventing a wide spectrum of disorders, including dementia.

Most of the recommendations we will be considering in this chapter fall within the *nonspecific* category. However, other suggestions may have some *specificity* to dementia. For example, some people have viewed Cayce's repeated warnings against aluminum toxicity as a *specific* suggestion for preventing Alzheimer's dementia. Therefore we will look at a variety of interventions ranging from extremely *nonspecific* (general health care suggestions) to relatively *specific* (aimed specifically at preventing Alzheimer's dementia).

The preventative measures which I am about to describe are also comprehensive. They may be helpful in preventing both "reversible" and "irreversible" dementias. They deal with the issue of genetic predisposition. They address environmental factors such as aluminum toxicity. Finally, they are holistic because they encompass all three aspects of the self (body, mind, and spirit).

A Holistic Preventative Plan

The following preventative recommendations are based upon the holistic approach advocated in the readings. We will discuss each aspect beginning with the physical dimension and then moving on to mental and spiritual suggestions.

Remember that the readings took a broader view of the causes and treatment of dementia than current medical science. The readings insisted that we consider the whole body, and particularly the relationship between the central and autonomic nervous systems. In terms of preventative measures, this translates into a consistent regimen of therapies and lifestyle choices that strengthen these key systems and make the body more resistant to dementia from any source.

In other words, many of the basic therapies which were recommended for the treatment of dementia may also help to prevent it. Most of these interventions (which were presented in earlier chapters) fall within the domain of basic health maintenance. The readings stated that certain treatments such as spinal manipulations, hydrotherapy, balanced diet, regular moderate exercise, and certain forms of electrotherapy would be good for everyone on a regular basis. These recommendations tend to be safe, natural, and relatively inexpensive. They address two key problems which the readings frequently linked to dementia and cited as necessary for effective treatment—coordination of the nervous systems and improved eliminations to reduce toxicity within the body.

Spinal manipulation was one of primary therapies recommended to address incoordination of the nervous systems and poor eliminations (see Chapter Three). The readings insisted that everyone could benefit from an occasional "tune-up," as it were. Naturally, the frequency of these treatments depended upon the individual's condition. A relatively healthy person who had no history of spinal injury might do well with a short series of treatments (for example, one or two treatments per week for two or three weeks). A couple of these series per year might serve to maintenance the body in a similar manner in which we take our automobiles for regular maintenance (such as rotating tires, tune-ups, etc.).

The concept of specificity and nonspecificity even carries over into the area of physical therapies. For example, the readings distinguished between spinal adjustments which were *general* (nonspecific) and *specific* treatments. A general treatment addresses the whole body and serves to coordinate or balance the nervous systems. The readings insisted that all persons could benefit from such treatments regardless of whether they were having any particular problem. *General* treatments also help to improve eliminations (thus reducing toxicity within the body).

On the other hand, a *specific* treatment focuses on a particular problem that needs correction (for example, a misalignment of spinal segments). In either form (general or specific), the treatments can serve to keep the nervous systems coordinating and help to prevent illness.

Of course, persons with more serious spinal problems may require more extensive "repairs." Even in such cases, the readings consistently recommended taking the treatments in series in which the body would be allowed to rest and re-establish equilibrium between each series of treatment. Such series often involved alternating between both *general* and *specific* types of treatments. He seemed to be telling the doctors to be kind to the body. Use common sense in making the corrections. Don't continually and exclusively focus treatment on a certain area of the spine in order to make a correction. Give it a rest by mixing in some general treatments and taking a regular vacation from treatments. For example, take the treatments for three or four weeks and then rest for a couple of weeks before attempting further corrections. This style of treatment is entirely consistent with the principle that all healing comes from within. Give the body a chance to heal itself—don't force the issue by overtreating.

If the concept of general and specific physical treatments is confusing to you, don't be discouraged. Even many health care professionals are unfamiliar with this approach to helping the body stay healthy. If possible, find a physician (whether it be osteopath, chiropractor, physical therapist, etc.) who is familiar with the Cayce readings. Such a person can assist you in implementing a program for maintaining coordination of the nervous systems by way of spinal manipulation.

The readings also insisted on the value of hydrotherapy as a preventative measure which would be helpful for everyone. Hydrotherapy simply means the use of water to regain or maintain health. Drinking an adequate amount of pure water is the most basic form of hydrotherapy. For most people, the readings recommended six to eight glassfuls per day.

Colonics were also highly recommended. The readings noted that it would be good for everyone to take an occasional internal bath from time to time. A colonic is a highly controlled bathing of the colon. Warm water (body temperature) is gently flushed through the bowels to remove wastes and cleanse the colon tissue. A colonic is similar to an enema, only more thorough.

The readings insisted that colonics be "scientifically" administered. Readers wishing more information on this form of hydrotherapy can contact local practitioners for a description of the process and cost of treatment. As a preventative measure, many people follow a quarterly pattern of colonic cleansing by getting a colonic four times a year at the change of the seasons. Other therapies such as diet and hot packs may be combined to increase the effectiveness of colonic irrigation.

Steam baths were another commonly suggested form of hydrotherapy recommended as a preventative treatment. A steam bath can become a "fume bath" if medicinal substances are mixed with the steam vapor. The readings often recommended natural solutions such as witch hazel, pine needle oil, and wintergreen oil to increase eliminations and thus help to purify the body.

A body rub (full body massage) was usually advised as a followup to the steam/fume bath. While the massage addresses the whole body, it can be particularly helpful as a means of coordinating the nervous systems. The readings contain many references to massage techniques and combinations of oils which may be beneficial to the nervous systems (as documented in *Edgar Cayce's Massage, Hydrotherapy & Healing Oils* by Joseph and Sandra Duggan; see the Appendix).

Getting a steam and massage is also an excellent form of stress reduction as well as a means of cleansing the body and coordinating the nervous systems. Once a week is ideal; once a month is still great, if your budget is limited. Also consider getting or trading massages with friends or relatives. Harold Reilly's book *The Edgar Cayce Handbook for Health Through Drugless Therapy* is another superb resource on numerous forms of healing, including recommendations for doing steam baths and massage at home (see the Appendix).

The Cayce material has long been recognized as a valuable resource on diet and nutrition. In regards to the relationship between diet and preventing dementia, the key word would probably be balance. The readings stressed the importance of maintaining a healthy pH balance by selecting foods that tend toward alkalinity. Fresh vegetables and fruits form the core of this balanced diet. Fish and fowl were preferred as meats while avoiding refined carbohydrates, fried, and highly processed foods. The primary Cayce recommendations have become so widely accepted by health advocates that they can hardly be viewed as extreme.

The readings frequently recommended combining various treatments to improve effectiveness. For example, here is an excerpt from reading 4003-1 which notes the advantage of combining diet and hydrotherapy to improve eliminations:

> . . . the eliminations need to be increased . . . This may be done in no better manner than by having colonic irrigations occasionally and by including in the diet such things as figs, rhubarb and the like. (4003-1)

The readings were also out front in their emphasis on regular moderate exercise. Walking was cited as the most beneficial exercise for most people. However, it has to be consistent—not just on days when you feel like doing it.

Whereas the readings' recommendations for diet and exercise foreshadowed mainstream patterns in the area of health maintenance, the use of electrotherapy has not found widespread acceptance. While the readings prescribed numerous forms of electrotherapy over the years, one particular appliance was preferentially advised as a preventative that would be good for everyone to use. This device was called the Radio-Active Appliance. Its creation predated the splitting of the atom and its name in no way reflected the use of radioactive materials as we know them. To distinguish this form of electrotherapy from other treatments which involve harmful radiation, it is sometimes called by different names including Radial Appliance and Impedance Device. It is currently available through manufacturers who have developed their own trademarked names for the appliance. Douglas Richards, Ph.D., and I have written a book which covers all aspects of the use of this appliance. Our book and a list of appliances manufacturers are listed in the Appendix.

The readings say that this appliance does not produce any energy of its own, it merely uses the body's own natural low electrical forces. According to the readings, it can help to coordinate the nervous systems and equalize circulatory patterns.

It is simple to use. Most people do not feel anything when using the device. I personally find it to be an excellent tool for stress management—when I use the device in the evening, I sleep better and feel more rested upon waking.

We could go more deeply into the nuances of the readings' views on physical measures of a preventative nature. I prefer to let the readers pursue this material at their own pace, if they so desire.

However before we leave the subject of physical modalities, I do want to re-emphasize the importance of coordinating the nervous systems. The readings repeatedly emphasized the effectiveness of physical therapies in improving memory and concentration by improving nervous system coordination. Memory and concentration are two important cognitive functions which deteriorate in persons afflicted with dementia. Specifically, spinal corrections, spinal massage, and electrotherapy were suggested to improve coordination between the nervous systems. Here are a few selections which link nervous system coordination with memory and concentration:

This is the same sort of condition that arises from, or through, the lapse of memory, the tendency for the body to appear at times to be dreaming, or to be visionary. These, of course, are pressures or short-circuiting as it were of the nerve impulses from the body. Hence the electrical vibratory forces should tend to enliven the connections as it were in the sympathetic nerve system and the cerebrospinal nerve system.

Hence the massages and the low electrical forces as has been indicated. (1361-2)

Q. How may I improve my memory?
A. . . . coordinating of the physical body with the mental body creates that which is commonly known as memory. An assistance to this will be found in the use of the Radio-Active

Appliance, which is well for everyone and especially good with this body. (416-9)

. . . the pressures produced through the system in the present upon the nervous system—DO influence the nervous system's connection between the cerebrospinal and sympathetic systems; especially in the areas where subluxations were caused or produced by the first forms of affectation—producing a disturbance that arises from the nervous system; as the conditions in which there is the inability of the PHYSICAL nervous force or CENTRAL nervous system AND the sympathetic or vegetative system to at all times coordinate.

This disturbs the body in its ability to recall or to remember immediately . . . (2164-1)

Q. How can I improve my powers of concentration?
A. When there is removed a great deal of that distress between the coordinations of the cerebrospinal and sympathetic system, these should come back to near normal reactions— and concentration will be easier for the body. (2771-2)

Q. What will improve my ability to concentrate?
A. This again is almost as indicated. For when there are those tendencies for the combativeness in the influence of activities that produce a drain upon the vitality of the body, these prevent the coordination between the cerebrospinal and sympathetic system . . .

Hence the cleansing of the system in the manner as indicated. (1063-1)

The common thread which runs through all these suggestions for preventive physical measures is their naturalness. They work closely with the body to optimize nature's own processes. Health is maintained from within—the body is helped to take care of itself. Thus they tend to be relatively safe and sensible precautions aimed at maintaining health. A healthy body is less likely to fall prey to dementia, particularly the reversible dementias which can result from imbalances within the body's systems.

Mental Strategies for Preventing Dementia

Just as one can maintain physical health through certain preventative measures, a person can reduce the risk of catastrophic illness by how he or she thinks. The readings repeatedly asserted that "mind is the builder." As previously noted, they acknowledged the biblical observation that "as a man thinketh in his heart, so he is." They were also quick to point out that "thoughts are real things."

In the area of health maintenance, the readings asserted the powerful influence which positive thought can have. Especially when such mental activity is integrated with some of the physical recommendations presented in the previous section:

Q. How can I increase my vitality and energy?
A. By using that which exists in the physical forces of the body.

Here, in these periods of physical development, come those tendencies to dream, to react to WAITING responses.

Now, set thyself to be the control, through thy mental self (for mind is the builder), and budget thy time—for physical development, physical relaxation, physical improvement, mental relaxation, mental taxation, mental improvements and spiritual ideals. And keep true to that budget ye set for thyself. So much time for this, for that. And this will bring a consistent reaction, yet may not become rote. For, as the budget is set, make the daily activities coordinate in thy daily life. Not only will the vitality and energy improve, but there will be much more FULLNESS in the life experience . . .

Q. Please specify what I can do to improve my thinking capacity?
A. Study that as just given. Exercise of the body brings strength and resistance. Exercise of mental activity brings resistance, growth and expansion. (1206-13)

In sum, the readings seemed to be saying that mind is the builder—what you hold in your consciousness you will meet in your daily life. Make the experiences of your life healthy by holding healing thoughts of self and others. Use your mental abilities to help structure your life in a balanced way. Exercise your mind as you would your body, if you would maintain health.

The Spiritual Dimension in Preventing Dementia

If we do not take a holistic view of life, and especially of health and illness, we can be misled into the limitations of materialism. This view accepts the premise that the physical dimension of life is primary to the human experience. Thus, illnesses such as dementia are primarily (if not exclusively) of a biological nature. For a person caught up in this philosophy, it can appear preposterous to claim that spirituality is a factor in the treatment and prevention of dementia.

And yet, from a holistic perspective this is not only a tenable position, but unavoidable. The same practical spirituality which was emphasized in previous chapters as necessary for treating dementia can help prevent it. In treating a demented person, the caregivers must apply spiritual truths. This is natural because a person so afflicted may not even be coherent enough to understand much less apply such principles. However, in a preventative mode, any person is capable of such application. Thus, living a purposeful life while manifesting the "fruits of the spirit" becomes a matter of choice. Do you choose to be patient, kind, gentle, and long-suffering towards others while you still have health? If so, you are more likely to maintain such a state.

The readings insist that spirit is the basis of life. All healing is essentially spiritual in nature. It makes sense that living a life grounded in spirituality is a strong preventative measure.

So, in practical terms, what does living a spiritual life come down to? The answer has been around for ages. The admonition of "Love God with all your heart and others as yourself" is the foundation of spirituality.

Our current fascination with "love and relationships" underscores the importance of this area of our lives. Certainly, love relationships come in many packages—parent/child, friendship, romance, etc. The spiritual dimension of relationship seems related to an understanding of the context of relationship.

For example, if we see ourselves as merely biological beings at a certain stage in an evolutionary process, our relationships will reflect that view. We may relate to others in terms of survival (personal and collective).

However, if we broaden our view to a holistic perspective, relationship takes on a different meaning. From the standpoint of the readings, we are all spiritual beings utilizing a physical body as a vehicle of expression. While in the flesh we are triune entities (body, mind, and spirit). The context of human experience is that of souls making their way through eternity, finding their way back to their source.

Relationship is why we are here—it's what we are about. It is fundamental to the purpose of creation and the meaning of life. The readings state that the creator desired companionship and the process of creation and evolution is the unfoldment of that desire.

The earth experience thus becomes a series of lessons to help us become better companions. The lessons vary according to our needs. Apparently, some of us need to learn from severe diseases such as dementia. Perhaps working on our lessons before actually suffering such misery could avert such an extreme educational experience.

The readings provide abundant suggestions for awakening to our personal spiritual heritage. Studying inspirational materials to open our consciousness to the divine pattern within was advised. Individuals were encouraged to seek God through whatever source they found meaningful. Not surprisingly, the Bible was highly touted.

Naturally, prayer and meditation are emphasized in Cayce's readings. Most important, however, is the application of spiritual truths on a daily basis—in relationship, whether relating to ourselves, others, or God (or a "Higher Power" by whatever name). This is the meaning of "fruits of the spirit" as discussed in previous sections. Patience, kindness, gentleness, long-suffering—these are the fruits of the spirit that make for health and contentment in any relationship. They make sense as a preventative measure whether one is concerned about dementia or merely want to experience a purposeful life.

Preventing Alzheimer's Dementia

The previous holistic preventative measures should decrease the chances of suffering from dementia of any type. In the case of Alzheimer's disease, the key to recognizing preventive possibilities lies in the awareness that it may be a threshold illness.

For example, many brains exhibit the neuronal abnormalities characteristic of Alzheimer's disease without the individuals actually suffering any clinically recognizable symptoms. This we know from post-mortom studies of normal and diseased brains. This has led many researchers to the conclusion that Alzheimer's disease is not an "all or none illness." There may be varying levels of nerve degeneration which do not become clinically significant until this deterioration manifests in the characteristic symptomology. This is such an important point that I want to cite a couple of sources to emphasize the significance of the threshold concept. Here is how William Check, author of the book *Alzheimer's Disease,* describes the phenomenon:

> Another interesting fact that scientists discovered is that virtually all of the changes characteristic of Alzheimer's disease are also seen, although to a lesser degree, in the brains of elderly persons who do not have the disease . . . Alzheimer's disease is a threshold phenomenon, which occurs when cell death exceeds a certain limit or threshold, rather than being a "unique condition" that suddenly affects the brain. (William Check, *Alzheimer's Disease,* p. 34)

Dennis Selkoe, writing in the November 1991 issue of *Scientific American,* uses a more technical description to illustrate the concept of threshold:

> Most of us who live into our late seventies will develop at least a few senile plaques and neurofibrillary tangles, particularly in the hippocampus and other brain regions important for memory. For the most part, the distinction between normal brain aging and Alzheimer's disease is quantitative rather than qualitative. Usually patients with progressive dementia of the Alzheimer type have moderately or markedly more mature neuritic plaques and neurofibrillary tangles than age-matched non-demented people do.

Because the brain degeneration associated with Alzheimer's dementia is also common in the brains of most aged people who do not suffer from the illness, what causes the deterioration to surpass the threshold in afflicted individuals? Could nervous system incoordination, improper eliminations, and other *nonspecific* factors be involved in the degenerative process? Could the preventative measures advocated in this chapter help to reduce the risk of surpassing the dementia threshold. Obviously, we do not have the answers to these questions at this time. However the possibility that Alzheimer's dementia may be a threshold phenomenon does indeed leave the door open to such speculation.

For example, since glandular dysfunction and immune system abnormalities have been linked to Alzheimer's dementia (see Chapter One), it makes sense that we might reduce the risk of this illness by strengthening these key systems. According to the Cayce readings, all of the preventative measures listed in this chapter do positively affect glandular and immune functioning. Conceivably, these measures could be preventative by fortifying these systems and raising the threshold of dementia.

Studies of heredity also suggest that Alzheimer's disease is a threshold illness. For example, researchers have noted cases in which one identical twin may suffer from Alzheimer's dementia at an early age, while the other did not manifest any symptoms for many years later. Since the brains and nervous systems of these individuals were apparently identical at birth, there may have been environmental factors that made one twin more vulnerable than the other. We have mentioned some of the possible environmental factors in previous chapters and we will examine one of them more closely now.

Preventing Aluminum Toxicity

The readings consistently warned against aluminum toxicity decades before scientific research raised the alarm in regards to a possible connection with Alzheimer's dementia. While many persons have directly associated Cayce's warnings about aluminum toxicity with Alzheimer's, after carefully looking over the material I cannot make such a direct assertion. The connection regarding general health maintenance is certainly there. I simply prefer to present a few excerpts on this subject and allow readers to determine for themselves whether this is something they want to pursue as a preventative measure against the risk of dementia:

> Do not use aluminum ware in any form where this body takes food from. (1223-1)

> Some it will never hurt to have prepared in aluminum, but in most people it gradually builds something not compatible with the better conditions in the body forces. This is with certain types of food. Those which are acid will take particles of aluminum into the body. (5211-1)

Where aluminum is used as the cooking vessels, and the food is directly in contact with same, there are produced those elements ever in the human system that become detrimental; unless there are certain characters of vitamins that make for the activity of certain glands in the body. In this body, as we find, there are certain traces; yet these having been changed or altered do not leave other than indications in the eliminating areas—as indicated. (445-2)

Q. Do I have aluminum or arsenate of lead poisoning?
A. Neither of these; though the effect of aluminum—or effect upon the body by foods being cooked in same—adds to rather than detracts from the activities in the system.
Hence, as we have indicated for many who are affected by nervous digestion or an overactivity of the nerve forces during the state of digestion taking place, the body should be warned about using or having foods cooked in aluminum. For this naturally produces a hardship upon the activities of the kidneys as related to the lower hepatic circulation, or the uric acid that is a part of the activity of the kidneys in eliminating same from the system. (843-7)

Note that these excerpts seem to indicate that not everyone is equally vulnerable to aluminum toxicity. This certainly is similar to Alzheimer's dementia where some individuals are at higher risk than others (for instance, due to hereditary factors).

There are so many forms of alternative cookware available it is not an extreme hardship for anyone to avoid this source of aluminum toxicity. Other aluminum sources are more subtle (such as stomach antacids, deodorants, and certain types of kidney dialysis). I think there is sufficient evidence in both the readings and the medical literature to cause a reasonable person desiring optimum health to avoid aluminum consumption as a matter of choice. If such a strategy also lowers the risk of Alzheimer's dementia, so much the better.

Genetic Vulnerability

The readings take a remarkable position with regards to hereditary factors and disease. Contained within the readings is the idea that the choices we make in our daily living can have an appreciable effect upon the unfoldment of genetic predisposition. The readings use the terms "hereditary tendency" and "hereditary innate" to differentiate the diversity of genetic patterns. Some patterns are merely tendencies—they will not necessarily play out in the development of the body.

Other hereditary patterns are perhaps biologically stronger—they are "innate" or inherent. Their effect is more certain—they must be dealt with in our life experience. The readings frequently associated this type of genetic influence with karma. The certainty that we will be offered the opportunity to meet our past actions is programmed into our cellular structure.

This view of heredity is congruent with modern medical research. Genetic patterns can manifest in a variety of ways, just as the readings indicated.

Since the readings stated that some hereditary factors could be influenced by preventative measures, this discussion is relevant to the subject of Alzheimer's dementia. Remember that this form of dementia is associated with a genetic component (Chapter One). Apparently the "genetic loading" in Alzheimer's is at least variable. That is, in some cases where there is a strong pattern of this illness in the immediate family background the probability that a family member will be afflicted is relatively high (yet not absolute). In other cases, the genetic pattern may not be so strong—perhaps indicative of a "tendency" rather than a certainty.

It is within the category of "hereditary tendency" that preventative measures have the most potential. There are at least two preventative measures specifically cited in the readings in such cases—mental patterns and the "vibratory metals." Let us look first at mental patterns.

The family of Mrs. [1873] were in a tizzy over her illness. She was suffering from a complex condition that was apparently approaching dementia. The readings stated that if the family got busy and implemented the recommendations:

> . . . we will bring a much nearer normal force and EVENTU-ALLY bring back to the activities of the body a balanced influence in the cerebrospinal and sympathetic [nervous] system—SAVING the brain itself. (1873-1)

The full range of treatment suggestions as discussed in previous chapters was recommended (i.e., manual therapy, electrotherapy with gold, etc.). However, the interesting aspect of this case lies in the possibility that her illness may have involved a genetic factor. One can almost hear the family members worrying among themselves about the possibility that [1873]'s condition might result from hereditary influences (in which case they might also be at risk). The reading noted this concern:

> And there should never be the impression or feeling (for others) that this is in ANY way a hereditary or prenatal condition, or one that would produce inclinations or weaknesses, or even tendencies in the lives or activities of others—UNLESS the mental selves of such individuals were to dwell upon same. (1873-1)

Pointedly, the reading cautioned them to stop worrying about it. Worrying could initiate a self-fulfilling prophecy, an example of the principle "mind is the builder."

Thus, it is possible that some genetic vulnerability may have been involved. That is, [1873] may have been genetically predisposed to suffer this illness. However, the genetic factor in itself was not enough to produce the illness. Some additional stressor was required to manifest the disorder (in this particular case a spinal injury was noted). In other family members, the stress of excessive worrying could perhaps trigger the genetic predisposition into action.

The idea of hereditary vulnerability combining with a stressor to produce disease is known as *diathesis/stress*—diathesis referring to a genetic predisposition and stress being any factor which triggers the inherited tendency into action. The stressor may be biological (such as a spinal injury, aluminum toxicity, brain insult such as "boxer's dementia," etc.); environmental (stressful life events); or psychological (such as worrying about inheriting the condition).

There are many such instances of *diathesis/stress* in the Cayce readings. For example, Mr. [282] suffered a psychotic breakdown (which the readings indicated was approaching softening of brain tissue or dementia). Family members were concerned that they might also be vulnerable since mental illness was known to have afflicted other members of the family. A sister (Mrs. [457]) was on the verge of a nervous breakdown. Being concerned that she might have inherited the condition, she requested Edgar Cayce's psychic assistance. Reading 457-4 states:

Q. Can I be in any way affected by it [the inherited condition]?

A. Only as the mental self dwells upon same and thus creates a field, an attitude for such reactions as to cause a disturbance. (457-4)

Reading 457-5 further cautions:

Do not dwell upon such. Be sure there is at all times sufficient Vitamin B in the diet, as well as with the blood test if found deficient in the procreative plasm then add same through the vibratory forces of Gold. (457-5)

The expression "mind is the builder" is actually presented here in quite literal terms. The "mental self" can actually create a "field" which manifests the undesirable hereditary pattern. The preventative measure in such cases is obvious—do not become obsessive in your thought patterns. Worrying will only increase the probability of its happening.

While it is easy to say to someone, "Stop worrying," it is usually much more difficult to apply such wisdom. In such cases, the best suggestion that I know of is to apply the recommendations in the earlier sections of this chapter which addressed the mental and spiritual aspects of prevention. In such application, most people develop the ability to constructively direct their mental processes to a significant degree. The spiritual influence is also helpful. Persons who awaken to their spiritual natures are less inclined to worry about any eventuality—even the possibility of dementia. As Cayce often counseled in the readings, "Why worry when you can pray."

The other primary preventative measure which was mentioned in both of the cases just cited was the use of vibratory metals—principally gold. This fits the theme of this whole chapter. Namely, that the treatments which are helpful for treating dementia may also be helpful as a preventative measure.

The application of this form of electrotherapy varies slightly with each individual—yet the principles are unchanging. Apply the treatments in cycles. Be gentle with the body. Be gradual in your applications. Be receptive to how your body responds to such measures and make adjustments accordingly. Maintain a positive attitude during therapy with the full expectation of good results. Be consistent and persistent.

The cycles of electrotherapeutic treatment need not be overdone. Furthermore, they are relatively safe and inexpensive. If Alzheimer's dementia runs strongly in your family, you may want to consider this measure. However, as with all of the suggestions in this book, individuals must decide for themselves upon the appropriateness of the information.

Summary

In this chapter we have considered a variety of preventative measures directed at maintaining health and decreasing the risk of dementia. As with previous chapters, the approach has been holistic—emphasizing the physical, mental, and spiritual aspects of health maintenance.

The preventative strategy outlined in this chapter is built upon a simple principle: the same applications used in treating dementia may also be helpful in preventing it. Or perhaps, to at least lessen its impact.

The foundation for this preventative approach was laid in previous chapters which focused on the importance of maintaining coordination between the nervous systems. Many of the applications fell within the category of *nonspecific* interventions which helped the body to do its job of maintaining coordination in these key systems.

We also considered some suggestions for persons at increased risk of suffering from Alzheimer's dementia. Specifically, a caution was given to avoid aluminum consumption. Furthermore, for those individuals at risk due to genetic vulnerability, we have discussed the importance of maintaining a positive attitude combined with the use of vibratory metals to assist in coordinating the nervous systems.

The preventative measures put forth in this chapter are relatively natural and safe. They are the type of activities which make for balanced living. In other words, they are likely to be beneficial regardless of one's vulnerability to suffering from dementia.

6

Summary and Conclusion

◆

IN CHAPTER ONE, we looked at the statistics and demographics of the dementias. They are frightening. Obviously, this is a problem which we cannot afford to ignore.

Undoubtedly, medical research will continue to make progress, thereby helping clinicians to understand and treat the dementias with greater effectiveness. However, given the track record of medical science in treating chronic, degenerative diseases, it is prudent that we should not close ourselves off to any plausible source of help.

I have attempted to present the Edgar Cayce information as one of the resources that can make a contribution in our attempts to address this serious problem. I have taken great care to present this material accurately insofar as keeping true to the content and intent of the readings. I have also taken considerable care not to "oversell" the potential of this perspective by making exaggerated or spurious claims. Rather, I have endeavored to walk the fine line of cautious optimism—of providing help and hope without disregarding the painful reality of the challenges which confront us.

In exploring this unpleasant subject, we have expanded the discussion beyond the suffering individuals stricken by dementia. We have considered some basic recommendations from the Cayce readings which each of us can consider as preventative steps. These practical interventions may lower the risk of suffering dementia. They also tend to be relatively natural and safe, falling within the domain of general health maintenance.

We have also gone beyond a mere biological analysis of the dementias and considered the mental and spiritual aspects as well. We have recognized the crucial role played by the beliefs and attitudes of caregivers. We have asked the question, "Why do you seek healing?" So that you may go on living as before? Or as an expansion in consciousness—a form of personal development which the readings identified as soul growth?

By raising these questions, the readings provided a framework for understanding the context of healing. Caregivers were challenged to set therapeutic goals and examine their expectations. Healing is not automatic for anyone. In some cases, the goal of treatment may simply be to delay or stop the deterioration caused by the dementia rather than produce an absolute cure.

We have acknowledged the difficulty of regenerating the nervous system. This is not a process that can be imposed on the body. Rather, such healing must come from within. We can only hope to stimulate healing by increasing the body's natural vitality and by providing constructive programming into its mentality by suggestion and example. The healing response must come from within the afflicted individual. In some cases this response may not come in any measurable way. There may not be any measurable physiological progress noted. And yet, from a larger perspective, there is always healing at some level when we reach out to help another person. The healing may be at a deep soul level. The healing may be within the caregiver.

In preceding chapters, we have briefly considered the numerous treatment options advocated in the readings. Based on these suggestions, one could put together a treatment regimen based solely on the Cayce material. Some persons may find such an approach worth the effort and decide to implement the information accordingly. Others may have questions and concerns which prevent such a focused effort. For such persons the possibility of an integrated approach is more plausible.

The Potential for Integration

While the readings tended to present a self-contained treatment plan for each individual, this information is not necessarily incompatible with mainstream treatment models. Although the readings generally avoided drugs and other medical interventions which worked against the body, there are many examples throughout the readings where the most powerful medicines and surgery were recommended for acute cases. Hence, caregivers may wish to consider integrating some of the suggestions from the readings into a comprehensive treatment plan for persons suffering from dementia.

As I mentioned in Chapter Two, the readings occasionally referred cases of dementia to institutions such as the Still-Hildreth Osteopathic Sanatorium. This institution was dedicated to the treatment of mental illness. Although there was no formal connection with Edgar Cayce, there was apparently a friendly association as Cayce made referrals over the years.

Apparently the treatment philosophy implemented at Still-Hildreth was very similar to the recommendations in the readings. In some readings making referrals to Still-Hildreth, there is little information given as to cause or treatment. The drift of these readings is simply that if the ill persons go to Still-Hildreth, everything that is necessary will be done.

The point is that the types of treatments consistently recommended in the readings can be provided in an institutional setting. Such care would probably not add much to the overall cost of operation and might make a significant contribution to understanding and treating dementia. In such a setting, the information from the readings could be integrated into an institutional model offering an optimal blend of natural remedies with the best of mainstream medical care.

Considering the number of nursing homes which presently serve as catch basins for society's demented elderly citizens, such a scenario may be plausible. A network of these facilities could make a notable contribution in dealing with the medical and social difficulties which are apparently before us.

Integrating the Cayce approach into an institutional model makes sense from a demographic standpoint. With the preponderance of two income households in our society, time and energy limitations and other family obligations make institutional care a primary option for treating demented relatives.

Problems with Implementing This Approach

There are two major problems confronting individuals wishing to implement Cayce's approach to treating dementia. First, there are not many health care professionals left who understand and apply the remedies recommended in the readings. Whereas practitioners of earlier decades were familiar with many of the therapies, most modern clinicians have adopted other approaches. This is particularly true with respect to the electrotherapeutic appliances recommended in the readings. In the early decades of this century, many, if not most, physicians routinely utilized such devices in their daily practice. Currently there is a much greater reliance on drugs as the intervention of choice.

In other words, there is no formal system for delivering many of the services discussed in this book. There are a significant number of knowledgeable and sincere health care professionals scattered around the country. There are also many dedicated lay persons who are attempting to apply this material. Interest seems to be growing. A network is forming. Case studies and research information are being shared among researchers and clinicians. It is a real grassroots movement at this point—its impact upon mainstream health care options remains to be determined.

Secondly, this approach is not for everyone. It is not being presented as a cure-all or therapeutic panacea. It can only be helpful to those individuals who are willing and able to invest the resources required for its implementation. Obviously, these resources encompass more than financial investment. Open-mindedness is an essential resource. The ability to hope—to have faith in the body's ability to heal itself; the vision to see healing occurring at more than the physical level; the sensitivity which recognizes and appreciates soul development in self and others—these are all valuable personal resources which must be invested in the healing process.

There are many who are unwilling or unable to make these investments. They would prefer to view dementia as a physical illness and let the medical system take care of the problem. However, even at this level an investment must be made. Such persons should seriously plan for the financial resources required to pay for these services. They should also support the research that will be necessary to provide even the hope of effective treatment. The investment must be made, one way or another.

Conclusion

Frankly, I am hesitant to present this material to the public. I recognize that many will find it difficult to seriously consider the work of a psychic diagnostician who died over forty years ago.

Nevertheless, the seriousness of the problem prompts me to make it available as a perspective for consideration. Not as a cure-all, not to arouse hope to an unreasonable degree, but merely for further consideration. I am prompted by the desperation of the demented victims and their families. I am prodded by the poverty of treatment options. Therefore, I present this alternative perspective with the hope that researchers and/or clinicians may be stimulated in a constructive way to look at this problem from a different angle.

Certainly, most mainstream researchers are not going to find it appealing. Yet, if only a few or perhaps even one individual finds this material useful, serendipity may strike again, as it has so often in the arena of medical research. Possibly this information could send medical science onto some productive yet unexpected path.

Realistically, one can more easily imagine such opportunities for research and clinical application on foreign soil where governmental and medical structures are typically more open to innovation. There is significant interest in subtle energy applications in Japan and the market for any breakthrough is certainly available. The restructuring of the Soviet Union also provides opportunities for alternative perspectives which require low investment and are easily accessible to mass application.

And of course, there is always the grassroots level of application within Western culture. Individuals may feel that they cannot wait for the medical establishment to find a cure. I suspect that this represents the most viable area of application of this material. Consequently, I have attempted to keep the presentation of this information as nontechnical and accessible as possible.

I have also published a treatment manual addressing the clinical application of the therapeutic principles and techniques presented in earlier chapters. Readers wishing to apply this approach should find it helpful. Health care professionals may also find it worthwhile (*Principles & Techniques of Nerve Regeneration: Alzheimer's Disease and the Dementias;* see the Appendix).

One final word on the application of this material. While the treatments recommended in the readings are relatively safe and inexpensive compared to mainstream medical options, individuals wishing to apply the information should seek the assistance and guidance of qualified health care professionals sympathetic to the perspective of the readings.

Appendix

◆

Association for Research and Enlightment (A.R.E.), 67th Street and Atlantic Avenue, P. O. Box 595, Virginia Beach, VA 23451-0595. Telephone (757)428-3588.

Baar Products, Inc. (distributor of electrical appliances and accessories which were recommended in the Cayce readings), P. O. Box 60, Downington, PA 19335. Telephone (215) 269-5059.

Bolduc, Henry L. *Self-Hypnosis: Creating Your Own Destiny.* Virginia Beach, Va.: A.R.E. Press, 1985.

Carroll, David L. *When Your Loved One Has Alzheimer's: A Caregivers Guide.* New York: Harper & Row, 1989.

Check, William A. *Alzheimer's Disease.* New York: Chelsea House Publishers, 1989.

Dippel, Raye L., & Hutton, J. Thomas (editors). *Caring for the Alzheimer's Patient.* Buffalo, N.Y.: Prometheus Books, 1991.

Duggan, Joseph & Sandra. *Edgar Cayce's Massage, Hydrotherapy & Healing Oils.* Virginia Beach, Va.: Inner Vision Publishing Company, 1989.

Heritage Store, Inc. (distributor of health products which were recommended in the Cayce readings), 314 Laskin Road, Virginia Beach, VA 23451. Telephone (757) 428-0400.

Home Health Products, Inc. (distributor of health products which were recommended in the Cayce readings), P. O. Box 3110, Virginia Beach, VA 23454. Telephone (757) 491-2200.

Karp, Reba Ann. *Edgar Cayce Encyclopedia of Healing.* New York: Warner Books, 1986.

McMillin, David L. *The Treatment of Schizophrenia: A Holistic Approach Based on the Readings of Edgar Cayce.* Virginia Beach, Va.: Lifeline Press, 1991.

McMillin, David L. *The Treatment of Depression: A Holistic Approach Based on the Readings of Edgar Cayce.* Virginia Beach, Va.: Lifeline Press, 1991.

McMillin, David L. *Principles & Techniques of Nerve Regeneration: Alzheimer's Disease and the Dementias.* Virginia Beach, Va.: Lifeline Press, 1995.

McMillin, David L., & Richards, Douglas G. *The Radial Appliance and Wet Cell Battery: Two Electrotherapeutic Devices Recommended by Edgar Cayce.* Virginia Beach, Va.: Lifeline Press, 1994.

Reilly, Harold J., & Brod, Ruth Hagy. *The Edgar Cayce Handbook for Health Through Drugless Therapy.* Virginia Beach, Va.: A.R.E. Press, 1987.

Selkoe, Dennis J. "Amyloid Protein and Alzheimer's Disease," *Scientific American* (November 1991).

The International Society for the Study of Subtle Energies and Energy Medicine (ISSSEEM). Central Office: 356 Goldco Circle, Golden, CO 80401. Headquarters and Business Telephone: (303) 278-2228.

Notes

Chapter 1

1. Dippel, Raye Lynne, and Hutton, J. Thomas, eds. *Caring for the Alzheimer Patient.* Buffalo, N.Y.: Prometheus Books, 1991.

2. Check, William A. *Alzheimer's Disease.* New York: Chelsea House Publishers, 1989.

3. Heston, Leonard L., et al. "Dementia of the Alzheimer's Type: Clinical Genetics, Natural History, and Associated Conditions." *Archives of General Psychiatry* 38 (October 1981): 1085-1090.

4. Tollefson, Gary D. "Short-Term Effects of the Calcium Channel Blocker Nimodipine (Bay-e-9736) in the Management of Primary Degenerative Dementia." *Biological Psychiatry* 27 (1990): 1133-1142.

A.R.E. PRESS

DISCOVER HOW THE EDGAR CAYCE MATERIAL CAN HELP YOU!

The Association for Research and Enlightenment, Inc. (A.R.E.®) was founded in 1931 by Edgar Cayce. Its international headquarters are in Virginia Beach, Virginia, where thousands of visitors come year round. Many more are helped and inspired by A.R.E.'s local activities in their own hometowns or by contact via mail (and now the Internet!) with A.R.E. headquarters.

People from all walks of life, all around the world, have discovered meaningful and life-transforming insights in the A.R.E. programs and materials, which focus on such areas as holistic health, dreams, family life, finding your best vocation, reincarnation, ESP, meditation, personal spirituality, and soul growth in small-group settings. Call us today on our toll-free number

1-800-333-4499

or

Explore our electronic visitor's center on the
INTERNET: http://www.are-cayce.com

We'll be happy to tell you more about how the work of the A.R.E. can help you!

A.R.E.
67th Street and Atlantic Avenue
P.O. Box 595
Virginia Beach, VA 23451-0595